Doctors Talking

Edited by

Hellen Matthews
&
John Bain

SCOTTISH CULTURAL PRESS
Edinburgh

First published in 1998 by

Scottish Cultural Press
14/130 Leith Walk
Edinburgh EH6 5DT
Tel: 0131 555 5950 Fax: 0131 555 5018
e-mail: scp@sol.co.uk
http://www.taynet.co.uk/users/scp

ISBN: 1 84017 030 1

Typeset by Neil Gowans

Printed and bound by ColourBooks Ltd., Dublin

Acknowledgements

This book is based on a series of taped conversations with GPs working in different settings in Scotland. There was no pre-determined set of questions: instead, each person was invited to set a context, reflect on her or his experience of general practice, and explore those issues that seemed significant. From that material the texts which follow were developed. Our warmest thanks go to the GPs who took part: without them, there would be no book. We are indebted, too, to the family of A— for their agreeing to the story of his death being included.

Thanks also go to the many people within the GP community in Scotland who took an interest in the project; in particular, we would like to mention David Blaney, who was much involved at the beginning, and David Snadden, who generously gave his time to discuss a range of issues and, in particular, contributed extensively to the introduction.

Finally, our thanks go to Rob Pogson for his photographs, to the staff of Tayside Centre for General Practice for their unfailing help and good humour in dealing with our computing inadequacies, and to Molly Russell for stoically committing to disc many, many hours of taped conversation.

Hellen Matthews
Aberdeen

John Bain
Dundee

Summer 1998

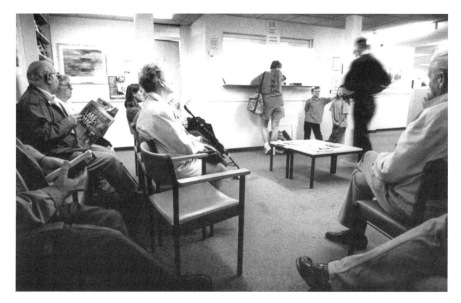

Waiting room

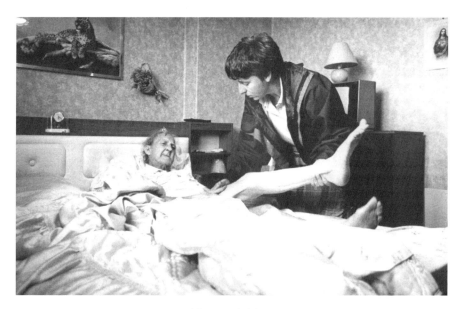

Home visiting

Introduction

General practitioners are part of the fabric of our lives, supporting our health and illness from infancy to old age. It's not so long ago that GPs or 'family doctors' delivered most of us into the world; in general they still see us out. Historically, in many communities – particularly in Scotland – the local doctor, often working single-handed, was a respected and influential figure, an educated person whose advice and expertise in dealing with many kinds of problems affecting people's lives and health could, in confidence, be sought. In terms of providing medical solutions to medical problems, however, the expertise of the general practitioner sixty or more years ago was actually quite limited, as there were few sophisticated drugs or treatments available to offer patients. Despite these limitations, however, GPs were widely credited with helping people back to health. Though we now know that much minor illness was and is self-limiting, the perception of the GP's role in recovery in the days before the technological explosion in medicine remains significant; it would seem a plausible explanation that the doctor's care, concern and empathy, and the patient's (and their family's) belief and trust in the doctor's healing powers, together created a powerful therapeutic instrument.

That people should have had such belief and trust is not so surprising when one considers how, fifty or more years ago, the same doctor might have delivered and cared for most or all of the children in a family, looked after the health of the parents, grandparents and other relations, and provided terminal care for those dying at home. Such continuing participation by one person in the major life events of a family inevitably forged, for many people, the sense of their GP as someone with whom they had a personal relationship; the value of this 'doctor–patient' relationship was recognised when, with the founding of the National Health Service in 1948, continuity of care became an established principle of general practice. This, in turn, served to further encourage the perception of a 'personal' service.

Fifty years on, the doctor–patient relationship still lies at the heart of general practice. Though it has often been perceived in the past as an unequal power relationship which takes its character from the patient's dependence on the doctor's expertise, in the 1990s it is, in reality, much more complex than this image would suggest. Many of the problems which patients bring to their GP have no straightforward solution, and, increasingly, doctor and patient must try to find ways forward together; the patient's environment, attitude and level of education, the particular interests and professional philosophy of the GP, and the personalities of both doctor and patient and the demands they consequently make on each other, all influence what happens. Because so much illness or lack of health is not separable from the context of patients' lives, much of the actual work of GPs connects as much with the historical and symbolic role of healers as with any ability to provide rapid cures. Such things as chronic illness, emotional distress and societal turmoil are as likely to take people to doctors these days as treatable disease processes.

General practice is about unorganised illness; unlike the specialist medical services, which come into play after a selection process has been applied to patients, the GP's surgery is the first port of call for a vast range of illness and problems. Because of the commitment to continuing care for the physical *and* mental well being of patients, as well as the tradition of free and open access, it is often assumed that a whole range of healthcare demands, physical and psychological symptoms, intimate details of relationships and problems of living can be legitimately presented to GPs with a freedom which is absent from dealings with other parts of the medical service. As a consequence of the GP's continuing perceived role as healer – medical expert, wise counsel and advocate – the demands made are so wide-ranging, and the boundaries of legitimate expectation so blurred, that at times the personal lives of GPs cannot but be affected by the job they do. The costs can be high. It is difficult for the doctor to strike the balance between getting close enough to patients to be effective in supporting them, but not so close as to be affected by their difficulties. If doctors are unable to keep some kind of professional distance from patients' life situations, stresses inevitably appear in their own professional and personal lives.

The practice of medicine, even these days, is not just about technical fixes; it is also about wisdom – about the application of knowledge to particular situations; about judging what is the right thing to do for a particular person at a particular time. But how can the modern GP, faced with the overwhelming growth of scientific know-how, develop the confidence and wisdom to judge accurately when the person opposite simply needs compassion and understanding, and when they need intervention of a technical kind as well? Modern medical journals are full of narratives of complaint and failure, but often, on analysis, it becomes clear that it is not technical prowess which has been at fault, but lack of communication, understanding and empathy.

Modern medical schools have struggled to bring a balance to the development of young doctors. With training often driven by doctors who are themselves pursuing a research-based agenda, there has sometimes been little in the curriculum to nurture the development and exploration of human caring skills, compassion and wisdom. Recent valiant attempts to change medical school curricula to encourage the development of these humanistic skills are to be applauded, because to become an effective generalist – a healer in the true symbolic sense – something else, apart from scientific training, has to happen to the would-be doctor. This may simply be a matter of the doctor being open and confident enough to learn from the patients themselves, sensitive enough to the lessons of experience and wise enough to include background knowledge of families and of psychology, in the widest sense, in the diagnostic and treatment armoury.

The healthcare reforms of 1990 introduced the concept of market forces to the NHS and ushered in a period of considerable upheaval; a new GP contract which focused on rewards for items of service and for carrying out questionable health promotion activities undoubtedly led to increased form filling for GPs and to concerns about excessive workload.

The other major innovation – the creation of a fund-holding system for general practice – was perceived by GPs in different ways. While some welcomed the new purchasing power as a means of developing services, others rejected it on the grounds that it created a two-tier system of access within the NHS in which the patients of fund-holding practices were immediately advantaged. This, the critics argued, undermined the principle of equality in the queue for treatment; they also took the view that it allowed medical care to be dominated by managers consumed by cost-effectiveness and the bottom line.

The election of a different government in May 1997 has led to further changes; these emphasise collaboration rather than competition between practices. Many GPs, however, remain sceptical about these changes too, perceiving in them threats to their cherished independence.

Fifty years after the founding of the NHS, it is perhaps timely to ask questions, not only about the training and function of GPs in our society, but also about what we might mean by health, health promotion and illness. In the chapters that follow, eleven of the 3,000+ GPs in Scotland reflect on their own working lives and offer a variety of insights into these questions. The impact of socio-economic factors on the work of GPs is huge; this is because the job is not just determined by training, though that provides a necessary knowledge and skills base; it is above all determined by the community of patients who walk through the surgery door, by their life circumstances and needs, their perceptions of health and illness, and their assumptions about what a GP is there for. We live in a society where problems of living seem to increase continually while traditional support structures in times of distress – such as the family and organised religion – decline. In this context, the 'healer' role of the GP comes under ever increasing pressure while the changing organisation of general practice makes the ideals of continuity of care and care for the whole person ever more difficult to sustain.

1

Female GP
Graduated 1978
Location: Health Centre in a deprived city area

It wasn't an obvious choice for me to become a doctor: I wasn't terribly good at science at school so I had to work really hard to get the qualifications I needed. But I've never been conscious of wanting to do anything other than medicine. I've also always wanted to do general practice – I like people, I'm patient and reasonably good at communicating with them, and I don't feel threatened by them.

General practice appealed to me because of the variety of work; even though I enjoyed all my hospital jobs, I never had any desire to stay in hospital medicine because I didn't want to be pinned down into a particular field. I also felt, and still do feel, that as a GP you have more freedom to make of the job what you will; in hospital medicine, even as a consultant, you're very much hedged about by administrators and other people telling you what to do and what use to make of your time. I think, though, that it's important to have experience in hospital jobs before you become a GP – to mature you as a person. Managing terminal care, for example, is not easy at first – knowing what to say to the relatives, knowing how to support them, can be more difficult than dealing with the patient. Equally, having the confidence to deal with children – handling small babies, coping with anxious parents – may only come when you've had children of your own. You understand parents' anxieties much better when you've experienced the anxiety yourself.

I was in a slightly unusual GP training scheme where I did 18 months in practice instead of the two years in hospital and one year in practice which people do now. Although I was in two inner city practices they were very different: I had six months in a very small practice, and then a year with a larger group. I found that arrangement very useful – it's a pity that at the moment registrars are not given the opportunity to experience more than one setting. Best of all would be to get experience of both rural and urban practice because the responsibilities are quite different. You get a bit lazy in a city because you know that help is always close by; if someone has a heart attack, for example, you can get an ambulance in two minutes. In a rural practice you have to carry all the necessary equipment for that kind of emergency yourself and you may also have to do much more in the way of resuscitation because it could take up to an hour for an ambulance to reach you.

The small practice I was in was very small – a husband and wife with a very low list, very low workload. I found it boring in a way. My other experience in a much larger group practice in a more deprived part of the city was far more interesting and I learned much more. It was more difficult in some ways because there were a lot of alcoholics (though not, at that time, a lot of people with other drug addictions), but the atmosphere was very supportive. You could go to different partners for help with particular problems – one was particularly strong on psychiatric problems, another on asthma and so on. I think it was there that I became clear about the kind of practice I'd like to work in – which is why I'm here.

There are six practices here – one single-handed and the rest all four or five doctors – in a Health Centre which has recently been renovated and which is owned by the Health Board. I'm in a practice of five and work a thirty-hour week. It's a fairly young group now, and quite forward-looking; we would like to become a training practice; that means that we would have a young registrar training with us. We have a community psychiatric resource centre attached to the Health Centre. It's mainly for long-term supervision of people who've left long-term care in hospitals, but we also provide support for people who are just not coping. There's assertiveness training and so on for people who are very lacking in confidence, very anxious. That's been useful. We have 6,500 patients from within the immediate area, mostly social class 4 and 5, though there's a smattering of social class 2 and 3. There's a lot of poverty, alcoholism, drug-addiction, and a large proportion of single mothers, increasing at the moment. There's quite a number of high-demand patients – regular attenders with up to three volumes of records!

Community care of older people is a big part of this practice's work; we've got district nurses, a geriatric nurse and a health visitor. It constantly surprises me how much people will put up with when they're looking after elderly infirm people before they shout for help – for example we have an elderly male patient in the practice who's looked after by his common-law wife even although she doesn't live in the house any more. He has very bad Parkinson's disease, is not really mobile, quite poorly and really requiring 24-hour nursing. Social work have been in touch but been turned away. Knowing the woman I was quite surprised at her caring for him but she's just like a lot of other people around here who think this is just their job and they're going to see it through despite poor housing, low incomes and so on.

Most housing round here is council and varies very much in standard. The older people with more points tend to live in the better housing. The worst areas, where it tends to be younger tenants, are horrible smelly closes that nobody cleans, smelling of urine and with syringes and crisp bags and things lying on the stairs – poor, worn carpets, second-hand furniture – quite dangerous if you have children. And yet up the same close you'll find immaculate houses where there's not any more money – it's just a question of priorities. Also, you'll find people coming in here clean and immaculately dressed and you can't believe they've come from such pits, and the reverse is also true. But people put on an effort to come to the doctor.

If things get out of hand with elderly people that can be difficult. I can think of two people that we've had to section under the Mental Health Act to get them into hospital. We can get the house cleaned up, but if they come back it takes a lot of support from home helps, social work and so on, to maintain them. They're usually people with vague psychiatric problems. We have one lady who's very obsessional. For a while she would only let one of our partners in to see her and her house was absolutely filthy. It's part of her illness that she hoards things. The house is full of toilet paper because she picks things up off the floor with it. She'll go through around a dozen toilet rolls in a couple of days, but she won't tidy up the house, so the home help has to sneak around getting rubbish out of the house. It's interesting to see these people – you can't let it upset you because you'd never survive if you did. I'd have to admit it's depressing at times though – a morning with depressed patients does rub off on you!

We have to work very hard to achieve our health targets here. My husband works in a practice in a middle-class area nearby with fewer doctors and a much bigger list, and their workload, including out-of-hours calls, is nothing like ours. A good illustration of our difficulties would be to compare the responses in these two practices to the offer of 'under age

2' immunisations. GPs are paid according to whether they reach 70% or 90% of their target group; in a middle class area you'll call the children in and get a 100% response first time; here we have to keep calling them up until they *are* 2 – call them eight or nine times – and even then we very often end up grabbing them if they're in for something else. So although we do reach our 90% target, the effort is enormous.

Prescriptions are also a big issue in this area. Whereas in a middle class area people will buy themselves things from the chemist, people here will come to the surgery for a prescription even for things like aspirin, paracetamol, nappy creams, because if you're on income support – as many of them are – it's free. They come for these prescriptions for a mixture of reasons; some patients genuinely couldn't afford the medication otherwise, but I'd have to say I don't feel very sympathetic towards people I know are spending £20–£30 a week on cigarettes and then claiming they can't afford paracetamol. I do point out that these medicines can be bought over the counter, and some people will respond, but a lot don't and say its their *right* to have a prescription. Very difficult!

I don't know what the answer is though. There *is* a poverty trap round here which you can't easily get rid of. It's undoubtedly related to a poor level of education – the majority of people have left school early with no qualifications. Hardly any children go on to higher education – they'd be made a fool of if they did. Most kids leave school at sixteen and – though obviously there are exceptions to the rule – the girls get pregnant and the boys get into drugs. In the past round here, if you were a boy doing really well at school, you would have got an apprenticeship in the shipyards or in a garage, but those jobs are gone, so the boys are unemployed and bored and get into trouble. I think they just see no future for themselves.

There's quite a widespread attitude of hopelessness about this area; you notice it when you're driving into the city. Five minutes away from here everyone's in employment, nearly everybody goes into higher education, it's all private housing. You come down here and you see people hanging about in the street with a gaggle of children around them because there's nothing else to do. They'll be smoking, grossly overweight and looking twenty years older than they should. It's very, very depressing – and this is not the worst area in the city.

As a woman doctor I have a very large proportion of female patients – not just with gynaecological problems but with psychiatric problems too. Stress is one of the main problems I deal with. GPs, on the whole, see a large proportion of depression and stress, only a small proportion of which is actually referred on to psychiatrists or psychologists. I see a lot of women beaten up by alcoholic husbands – it's one of our worst problems. We do have some women who are heavy drinkers or have drug problems, but alcoholic men are *so* difficult to deal with – the violence is *always* related to drinking. The women come in for a tranquilliser to help them cope with an aggressive partner or they come in for anti-depressants to help cope with the stress of financial problems, and you're aware even as you're writing the prescription that this is not the answer. It's a panacea, and really what they need is a solution to the problem, but there isn't always one available. You can refer the couple to marriage guidance, to social work departments, but very often they won't go and there's really no other answer.

We've a far higher proportion of patients on tranquillisers than we should have, but when you look through the records you realise it's the only thing that makes life bearable for them. It's particularly difficult for women if they have a young family and really have nowhere else they could go, because they know nowadays they can't get a council house easily. For that they would have to be declared homeless and enter a homeless unit for a while, but many don't want to inflict that experience on their children, so they stay with the husband until the children grow up and then, quite often, they just leave. But meantime they've spent fifteen, twenty years of their lives being regularly knocked senseless. Often the wife will say that the husband's fine when he's sober and keep on forgiving him, going back to the situation, but then she's down seeing us the very next day after he's beaten her up again, and so it goes on and on and on.

These women's lives are sort of ritualised. You get the crisis phone call around 5 o'clock in the evening, or the woman comes in around 5.30 with a black eye, clutching the baby, saying they've been thrown out. By that time you have to find emergency social workers, so you spend half an hour on the phone trying to get through, social work takes them into a homeless unit for the night, but the next day they're away back home and the whole pattern begins again. I think this lifestyle does affect the children. It's very bleak for me, too, as the doctor – very depressing. You know you don't have the answers and equally you don't know who else has. I can see that if the woman was working she'd have some income and could get a house of her own, be able to pay the rent, but she can't do that because she's poorly educated and can't get a job. So she's stuck in the house with the children and a violent partner – stuck just like women a generation ago were stuck because she has no means of her own. Some things haven't moved on in this area at all – it's very bleak – but worst of all these women know what the man is going to be like. I can't believe how these girls get beaten up by a guy when they're pregnant and *still* marry him.

The girls that have started off as single mothers are sometimes in a better position; they've managed to get benefits, they're used to living on their own. True, the boyfriends come and go and maybe give them another child, but they're much more independent. A lot of these girls would have done quite well if only they hadn't got pregnant so young – many of them haven't achieved their potential intellectually. And some of them are super with their children – keep them really nice, want them to go to a decent primary school and so on. I think the baby clinic maybe helps – they come in and see how other mothers from different backgrounds handle their children, and they listen to what goes on – listen to the health visitor, take in a lot too from television and the papers. One of the health visitors who has been here a long time is like an auntie to them; they trust her. Having said that it's also true that a lot of children around here are being brought up in a pretty uncaring sort of way. Some of them are rather hyperactive; they have no routines, they're going to bed very late at night, moving from house to house, never in one area for any length of time. When they're a bit older it shows up in criminal, almost psychopathic, behaviour; stealing and breaking into cars even at age nine or ten. Quite a few kids that age have been arrested breaking into cars in full daylight when people can see them; it's almost as if they're wanting attention. There are little pockets around this neighbourhood where you wouldn't leave your car unguarded for a moment because the kids'll break into it as soon as you've got out. Those areas are ghettos – the police won't go into them.

Apart from women patients, a lot of my work is with young families. There's a lot of low-level childhood illness here – coughs and colds for example. Parents have the idea that an antibiotic will cure everything and there's an educational job to be done explaining to them that it's not necessarily appropriate. A lot of the demand for appointments for children comes, I think, from the fact that we have so many lone parents without the supports there used to be. There's no granny living nearby to lean on for advice any more – because granny may well have a young family of her own – so the child is brought to the doctor. There's a widespread lack of advice and support and a lot of ignorance; a lot of these young mothers, who are just young girls, get so frightened if the baby is unwell and they don't know how to cope. I feel quite sympathetic to them, so I try not to shoo them away even if I'm a bit harassed. I feel if I can explain to them what's going on and what to look out for they'll gradually *learn* to cope, and manage the next child better. It's really an educational process, but you're talking ten, fifteen years before you may see the benefits.

The only place where the role of granny is still intact here is in Asian families, who make up about 8% of our list. On the whole these families don't bother us because granny sorts them out. She's usually on the ball, quite good, quite sensible as long as we can understand each other. There's always a communication problem with Asian grannies because they stay at home and are not well integrated. They look after the grandchildren and the daughters are made to go out to work in the shop, so the children are actually separated from their mothers at quite a young age. Sometimes the power of granny can be quite a problem. We have one family where an English–Asian girl who'd made an arranged marriage came up here and was completely miserable. She was a nurse – a well-educated girl – but she was told in no uncertain terms by her mother-in-law that she couldn't stay at home with her children; she had to go out to the shop while granny brought them up. The girl was really broken-hearted because she hardly ever saw her children awake. She's now left her husband, taken the children with her and got a job as a nurse again. She's been ostracised by the Asian community because of what she's done, but she's so much happier now. She has to have childminders looking after the children while she works, but she feels she has so much more control over her life. I think there are going to be more and more problems of this kind with Asian families as younger women become more westernised and want to assert their own ideas.

Older Asian ladies take up a lot of appointments. Apparently their culture doesn't recognise depression (they don't have a word for it), so of course they convert their depressive symptoms into physical symptoms – vague aches and pains and so on. And they won't go out the door without a prescription to justify how they're feeling. In many cases the women are actually homesick; they want to go back to India because they haven't picked up the language or are being badly treated by their husbands, but they can't tell you that. If you ask them if they're feeling down, they just look at you blankly, but they're really getting painkillers for emotional pain, so it doesn't solve their problem. That's part of a pattern for GPs here – dealing with the very real problems of living that people have.

Your only way of doing your best sometimes is to 'medicalise' people's problems, because you're not allowed or not able to address the real problem. Asian women will not go and see a social worker for example whereas with the native Scottish population round here *everybody*'s got their social worker – it's almost a status thing! 'Who's *your* social worker?' Nobody's bothered by it. But with Asian women it may take several courses of tablets – which don't work – before they'll admit that the problem really needs the support of a psychiatrist or a psychiatric nurse. There are community centres in the area – we have a Chinese one too – and they at least give the women some social contact. People who go to them feel they're quite relaxed: you see the Asian women all cheerful and uninhibited chatting away in their own language, whereas the rest of the time they're downtrodden and silent.

The language thing can be quite difficult when these older women come with physical ailments. Quite often they'll bring a grandchild to translate for them – but you can imagine what that's like if they come with a gynaecological problem and bring a young boy! It does limit the amount of information I can get. A lot of Chinese women have similar language problems, but they seem to be much tougher in some ways. We have a very small number of Chinese patients and they have a lot of contacts within the city so that helps. One of the worst problems for Asian women is moving away from their tenement community. The family makes a bit of money and wants to move out to a bungalow in a pleasant suburb. They get the dream house but they're more isolated than ever; they miss all the Asian shops and so on and they're surrounded by white people who look at them a bit more because there are fewer of them in the neighbourhood. Here white faces are in the minority in some streets!

I mentioned trying to educate our patients. To some extent we've been influenced by Health Promotion which gives us guidelines and targets each year – gathering data and so on. Smoking is one of our biggest problems. We have so many patients with chronic bronchitis and lung cancers which are smoking-related, so we try very hard to give advice about smoking. Diet and exercise are the two other big issues. The diet round here is generally pretty awful – a lot of high fat food. You only need to look down the main road – you've got chip shops and pizza shops and Chinese takeaways and curry houses. A lot of people here just live on carry-outs. One of my colleagues, who's a cardiologist, did a talk for us recently and took photographs of certain shops down the road. It suddenly brought it home to you just how many high fat food outlets there are in the area. You ask patients if they eat fruit and they look at you blindly. Fruit does not go down well here! You try to give advice and actually the men – with smoking – are paying more attention now than the women. We recently took part in a study which looked at the heart condition of populations in different parts of the country and it emerged that this area has the highest incidence of ischaemic heart disease in the country, worse with women than with men, and directly related to smoking and to cholesterol levels – which were related to some extent to the diet. Within the study population this area was actually the worst in Europe – which is pretty frightening!

It's been shown that the biggest influence on children smoking is whether or not their parents smoke, so it's self-perpetuating to some extent – very depressing. People are not motivated to stop even if you give them the statistics on bronchitis and cancer. They see that as being in the future, and it doesn't mean anything to them. There's a very fatalistic attitude here: if they die they die. So many people around them die at 50 so they see it as a bonus if they survive longer. It's absolutely amazing. We have one family with an incredible history: the mother died at 42 having had both her legs amputated because of vascular disease caused by smoking. She eventually died of gangrene which worked its way up her body and they just kept chopping bits off her legs until there was nothing left to chop off. She continued to smoke like a chimney. Her sister who was also a heavy smoker had a blocked aorta and had a graft done in her mid-30s. This caused her so much anxiety that she increased her smoking to 60 a day, got lung cancer and died before she was 40. *All the children smoke.* You say to them: 'Look, if your mum and auntie hadn't smoked so much they'd be alive now'. Their reply is that it's obviously inherited so there's no point in stopping. 'If we get it we get it!' I don't know what you can do with them. I'd have thought an experience like that would have frightened anyone enough.

I find the fatalistic attitude very difficult. That's the big difference between here and a middle-class area where people will do their utmost *not* to die at 50 – or even much later! The reaction in an area like that is that, if someone you know dies of heart disease, you're down at your doctor right away having your cholesterol checked, getting your angiogram done to ensure you're alright. Not here. They've seen it all at first hand and still they won't stop. The number of young girls who smoke is very worrying – I'm sure that's why so many of them look much older than they are. I know several girls in their twenties who look like 50 – grossly overweight, skin all dried up and wrinkled, half a dozen kids so their figure's gone as well. Not a lot to look forward to I suppose.

All this neglect of yourself makes it difficult for us to get these women to come for screening and so on. A lot of women don't go for smears, breast-screening – anything like that. We've taken to sending a series of letters to get them to come in. The third letter really puts the frighteners on them. It spells out what cervical cancer does to you. *That brings them in.* But they'll still say when they come in: 'That was a terrible letter you sent me doctor!' and I think, 'Well, at least you're here!' Once they've had one smear and a full health check they will come back, but it's such a struggle the first time. The younger girls are not a problem because they know we'll not give them the Pill unless they come for a smear. The Family Planning Clinic does the same, so they know there's no escape. You need to get them young enough and get them into the habit. It's the older women again who are the problem – a little core between 50 and 60 years old who've had their family and don't need contraception, and they're quite embarrassed about being examined. Girls who are 20 now have very different attitudes to their bodies, to sex and so on, from women in their 50s and 60s. Some older women get into quite a state about being examined, and because they're so tense that of course makes it painful.

That in turn confirms their belief that it's an unpleasant examination and they resolve not to come back.

I do deliberately scare patients at times: we've had two women in the last year with cervical cancer, one of whom had not seen a doctor for 20 years. She wasn't even registered with anybody, and she just came in one day with advanced cancer of the cervix. She claimed she'd only had symptoms for 'several months' but I don't really believe that. This was just a woman who never went to a doctor or dentist. When I said to her, 'Look, you're going to have to see someone very quickly – you're going to need an operation – this is very serious,' it still didn't click with her what was going on. I didn't actually mention the word cancer but I did stress how serious it was – that she'd need extensive treatment – and it *still* didn't click! And we had another case like that – a woman who'd been sent repeated letters asking her to come for a smear for years – and she presented with weight loss and bleeding and advanced cancer. She knew herself what it was and had endured it for several months before she thought to come and see anybody.

It's hard being a doctor confronted with situations like these. I just feel angry. There are very few illnesses we can actually prevent or do something about, but cervical cancer *is* one of them. I admit I sometimes take my anger out on the patient a bit – which I shouldn't do – but I make it clear to them that I feel they should have come earlier. It really annoys me when something's preventable. It's such a waste!

Interestingly, the attitude to breast lumps is different – they're down here like a shot with breast lumps. Not the very old ladies though (women in their 80s will hang on to them until they're actually fungating through the skin), but very elderly women usually do quite well because of their age. They don't usually require surgery; they get tamoxifen, a hormone treatment for breast cancer, and that usually helps them – and they can survive a good while. The difference in attitude to these two problems is interesting. I think there's been more publicity about breast cancer – high profile actresses in soaps having it and so on – and also women can't see their cervix, often don't know where it is. From time to time, too, there's a lot of bad publicity about inaccurate cervical smear results, which doesn't help. There's a lot of anxiety about the results, even if there's no reason to be suspicious – no history of suspect cells. Research in Aberdeen showed that a cervix shown to be healthy when a first smear is taken is more likely to go on being healthy – and it is anyway a slow-moving disease, so you've plenty of time to catch it.

I think breast screening can lull people into a false sense of security however: once every three years is not a lot. Breast cancers can develop rapidly – appear within months. The difficulty there is trying to persuade women to examine their breasts regularly. We have patients who come down here every three months for breast examination because they can't bear the thought of examining themselves, and they obviously have this thing about any part of their body. It's cultural I think – a real inhibition among older women about touching your body or talking about it. Young women are different; they take more pride in their appearance and so they think about things like breast lumps – and they're more likely to talk to each other. We have a women's centre down the road where they run groups that discuss health and exercise and so on. You quite often find someone coming in because of something they've been alerted to down there. Even the older women are beginning to get involved: there's an over-50s fitness club now too, but the problem's motivating people to go. And a lot of older women are trapped by being carers of demented relatives and so on, so they don't feel they've got the time to take part.

It's an ambiguous role being a GP – it's formal but it's intimate. I think how you do the job depends a lot on your personality and on the personality of the patient. Patients have interesting strategies sometimes when they have something very intimate to reveal – about having been abused, for example – which they would find *more* difficult to talk to you about because you know them well. So they'll go off and tell one of your partners about it, but then it's there in the notes for you to read and the next time you see them you will know, and they'll know you know, but they haven't had to tell you, don't need to discuss it with you. And if you then, for some reason, raise it after that they're quite relaxed about it, because it's already out in the open; but they couldn't have told you face to face.

General practice has changed so much. Before the 1990 contract I'd have said that the best things were just seeing patients and making diagnoses, but there's less of that now. A lot of the enjoyment's gone out of the job. The bureaucracy is awful. Our workload has increased because patient demand has gone up. Because of all the publicity about the health service they now expect more of us clinically, but the paper work is still the worst thing. However, I still think the freedom and the relative autonomy we've got is important; despite targets and all these other things, we can still make our working day and decide what our priorities are within the practice. I also like the variety there is in general practice and I enjoy seeing patients in their own environment – that's so much more enjoyable than a sterile hospital situation.

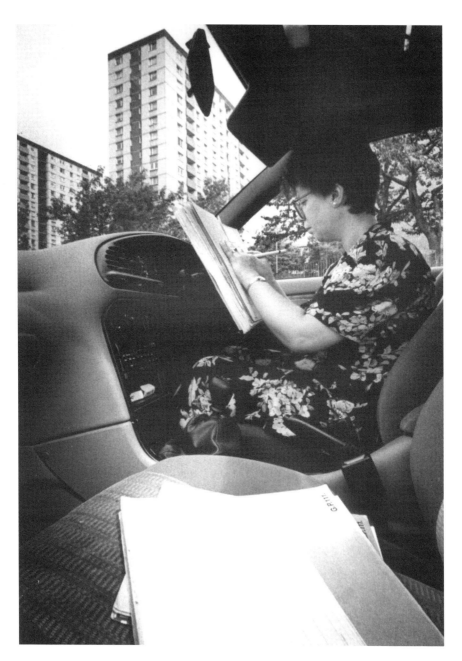

Housing estate visits

2

Male GP
Graduated 1978
Location: Group practice, affluent city area

Why did I become a doctor? I suppose the single greatest influence was that my father was a surgeon, but also, for people like myself who are now in their forties, if you did well at school you tended to do sciences and if you did well at sciences you tended to do medicine. So I suppose, to be honest, I really drifted into it – a passive rather than an active choice. The decision to go into general practice was somewhat different: I originally trained in surgery, and while I enjoyed the technical challenge, there was no doubt in my mind that it was the actual dealing with people that gave me most pleasure and satisfaction. So after several years in surgery I went into general practice, because of the opportunity to be involved with people on an ongoing basis.

I've always been in this practice, and we've changed very deliberately during the time I've been here. When I first came there were three male doctors and 5,400 patients: we're now five doctors – three males, two females – serving just under 7,000 patients. Recruiting female partners came simply from a recognition that female patients prefer to see them; but we try to be much more proactive now by anticipating things that patients want, as well as meeting their needs. Giving people access to good premises, practice nurses, competent doctors who are themselves in different age-groups, are all very important aspects of providing a quality service. We've made a deliberate effort to enhance the surgery premises so that people take pride in it, and feel we're taking care of them, making the effort to create a pleasant place for them: the days of the lock-up are hopefully long gone. In terms of the feedback we get the patient satisfaction levels are very acceptable – and then there are other vaguer indicators: one of the marvellous bits of general practice is Christmas – it's really very humbling, patients bringing presents. We get a marvellous supply of shortbread and biscuits!

We're a socially split practice in that we have a large number of social class 1, 2 and 3 patients, though we also take in a fairly large council estate which is very much more social class 4 and 5 – but generally this is a relatively affluent area. The practice is quite unusual in that we have an enormous number of older patients; that's to do with the neighbourhood, which grew up as an extension of the city in the 1930s. Many of our patients moved in then, and 60 years on they've gone from 30 years old to 90: we still have many patients who are only the first or second people to stay in their house. As elderly people move away, younger families move in, so we're unlike most city practices in that our population's growing rather than shrinking; but we do have a lot of elderly people still, and increasing numbers of nursing homes and residential homes in the area.

The high proportion of elderly patients changes our workload dramatically. Instead of having large numbers of children with infectious diseases, we have an enormous number of older patients with wear-and-tear and degenerative diseases. That means that instead of short-term acute episodes which younger people get, you're dealing with long, on-going situations: you don't cure arthritis, you try and control it; you don't cure heart disease, you try and control it: the focus is much more on trying to improve the *quality* of life. In that situation you can do much more by being proactive than by waiting till problems arise: for example, we can either wait until somebody of 85 living at home isn't coping and then try and sort out what we can do or, as we have done instead, we can put additional resources into community and practice nurses which lets us screen the elderly and identify what additional assistance they would benefit from – is their mobility deteriorating? – would physiotherapy help? – are there some aids that they could use at home which would make a difference? That's not in the traditional image of the NHS, which was coming to see the doctor when you were ill.

Screening and putting in resources has made a very big difference, but the knock-on effect in terms of appointments is awesome. In 1984 when I joined the practice, we had a list size of 5,400, and just over 12,500 appointments at five minute intervals. By last year, our list size had gone up by a quarter, but instead of 12,500 appointments we had *27,000* at *10* minute intervals, double the number of appointments and double the amount of time spent on each, so that's four times the amount of time that needs to be available.

The pressure to do more with the same resources is clearly affecting recruitment to general practice: people can see the incredible increase in workload, and patient expectation is much higher too, and ever-increasing. It's one of the lovely ironies of life at the moment that the population is healthier than they were 10 years ago – than they were 30 years ago – and yet they consult doctors much more regularly and everybody wants to be seen *now*, the same day, at a time convenient to *them*! I think the media has a lot to answer for here: scaremongering is a real problem. For example – everybody knows about meningitis, and while a GP will probably see one case of the killer type every 10 years, every week we have people coming in concerned about it. It's all to do with children: there's much less confidence around than a generation ago. I think that's partly due to a change in the family unit, in that there used to be granny in the background who could be phoned up for advice. Granny was the wise woman who would get the child's temperature down and do all the basic things before a parent would think of involving a doctor. Now, in an affluent area like this where mum and dad both work, what not infrequently happens is that they come home to find that the child has not been well with the nanny or in the nursery or whatever, they feel they must take the child to the doctor, and it must be that night. This partly springs from parental anxiety: they've been out at work, they lack knowledge of their own child, they lack confidence about what they're doing and so on – a combination of factors. It's certainly made a big difference.

There is considerable pressure on women who work. They have the impossible task of trying to marry everything – holding down a job, running a home, looking after children, juggling the most impossible set of demands. They're doing everything women did in the past plus a full-time job, and the pressures on them are very difficult – and that's reflected in having a lower threshold for shouting for help, looking for reassurance.

People living on their own also generate a lot of concern. With elderly people, their children get concerned: we increasingly have the problem that a lot of late 80s, early 90 year-olds live at home, and their children (who are 65 and 70) are not sure what to do if the parent becomes confused – they're unsure whether the parent can cope at home, so doctors get frequent calls late in the day or in the evening asking for something to be done. It's difficult, too, if the family feel that the elderly person should be removed to a safer place, while she or he wants to go on staying at home. We meet this all the time: the 60 year-old saying, 'Something's got to be done!' and the old person saying 'I don't want to go!'

When I trained as a GP many of the important things that we need to know about now weren't there. I think the Training year in General Practice is good, but they don't teach you about the financial side of running a practice, or about personnel management issues, never mind the more complex issues of how social work departments fit in, or what crisis care and care in the community are, or what the relevant legislation is. When I was a child, I can remember my own GP having just a receptionist – who was his wife! That still goes on, but we're much more of a unit here with practice nurses, community nurses, health visitors, reception staff as well as a number of doctors who cross-cover and exchange information about patients. You rely on working together much more, and so a considerable amount of time is needed for meetings. And organising health checks is very time-consuming. If we are to write to every woman who should have a cervical smear, we have to identify the patients, compose a letter that will be appropriate to a whole range of women of different ages, decide how to send the letters out so we don't have everyone turning up at once, and co-ordinate the availability of female doctors, practice nurses and so on. We also need to ensure that anyone with an abnormal smear is automatically followed up, and not just by computer. All these planning processes have to be repeated for a variety of health checks: we have, for example, more than 700 patients over 75 who are supposed to be screened annually – so that's two appointments a day for every day of the year, irrespective of public holidays, weekends and everything else. We also screen women for post-natal depression, and that means sitting down and going through a number of issues with each person. That, too, can be very time-consuming. And all this is just health promotion – nothing to do with the illnesses that are presented to us.

Because we run a fund, we're accountable for the taxpayer's money, so we set priorities and identify how we are going to try and implement them. There are national priorities (currently cancer, coronary heart disease, hardening of the arteries and mental health), so we try and integrate these with our own priorities for the practice in a way which will actually benefit the patient. There's an issue of resources here: where is the resource to come from? For example, if we're going to provide enhanced facilities for our elderly at home with new community nurses, how do we release the money to fund that?

One of the ways that we can release funds is by developing a strategic plan for how we use drugs; it's possible to be a bit idiosyncratic and innovative with prescriptions without altering patient care, and the money saved can be used for other projects. For example, though you prescribe a seven day course of antibiotics, the vast majority of patients only take them for five days, because by that time they're usually feeling better. If we therefore give them only five days' medication – if it's not clear we should be seeing them again anyway – we cut two-sevenths of the cost. For each individual prescription that's maybe not a lot but it fairly adds up. You might think there could be another cost, of course, in the patient having to come back to us, but the number that do is inordinately small.

Even more innovative is this: instead of giving my patient an NHS prescription for drugs like penicillin, common pain-killers and so on, which actually cost substantially less than the prescription charge, I can write a private prescription (if they prefer it). They will then pay only the cost of the drug plus a dispensing fee and the drugs won't cost our practice anything – a win/win situation. The practice can divert the money saved to fund other services – community nurses, cataract operations, a hip replacement perhaps. And you can motivate people with these economies because you can show the benefits.

The contentious topic in medicine at the minute is rationing, but in fact we've been rationing for years. We have choice on how we ration however; we can either restrict the number of people who get the service at all, or we can ask whether the treatment is going to be really effective in a particular case – providing a hip replacement for somebody who's 18 stone is less likely to be effective and lasting because they're so heavy; cardiac by-pass grafts for somebody who smokes 30 a day are almost certainly going to clog up within six or nine months; the key issue is how we apply the resource and who is prioritised.

Historically we've rationed hip replacements by saying, 'Here's an orthopaedic service, take your turn in the queue': what we're doing in this practice is slightly different. If we have a patient living in a nice affluent area down the road who can afford to take a taxi into town for lunch with her friends and back again, so that although she has severe arthritis she's not housebound, and there's also a lady who stays on the second floor of a tenement whose arthritis isn't as bad on x-ray but she *is* actually housebound because she can't get up and down the stairs, we'll put the lady from the tenement ahead in the queue for a hip replacement. It's looking at things in a more global way: if you take the decision-making closer to the patients it works. Prioritising is not about withholding treatment from anybody; it's saying the need for getting treatment sooner is here rather than there. Equally, we have never refused a drug to anybody *if it works*: we have several patients on growth hormone costing £12,500 a year. That's not a problem: we're able to find the £12,500 by making economies elsewhere. What is debatable, however, is whether patients with multiple sclerosis should be given the new beta interferon drug costing £10,000 a year when the evidence is that it may prevent one patient having on average one relapse every two years, but won't alter the course of the disease, or its severity, or the outcome. I would suggest that spending the £10,000 to treat, say, fifteen patients with cataracts instead, would give greater benefit.

If someone comes asking for something for which the research evidence is not strong, we try to inform the patient and discuss the issue with them. We had a very interesting situation about choices recently when the local health authority, which had not been purchasing IVF treatment in recent years, decided that it would put a small amount of money into it, enough to treat one patient out of a 7,000 population this year, and one in 14,000 next year. We identified all the patients who are on our waiting list for IVF treatment, and asked them whether they would wish us to nominate *one* patient to receive *all* the cost of the treatment (drugs and hospital costs), while everyone else got nothing, or whether, without knowing where they were in the queue, they would prefer us to give *everybody* the cost of the drugs *only* for as many cycles as they wanted, while they themselves met the hospital costs (which admittedly are greater). In this way we would be giving everybody on the waiting list some support and spreading the resource more widely. Every one of our patients said they'd rather that everybody had a helping hand.

One of the emotive issues in the philosophy of medicine at the moment is whether (even if we're all agreed that the NHS is under-funded) spending more is the way to make a difference to health. You'll certainly get happier doctors and nurses who are being paid more, but will you get healthier patients? In Scotland we spend 15% more per head of population on health than in England and Wales and yet in Scotland we die younger than they do in England and Wales and we are iller. A very provocative argument is that if you really want to improve people's health you don't spend more on the NHS – where you're always fighting a rearguard action – but put the money into employment and education instead, on the grounds that if you give people a job they will live longer and they will be healthier than if you simply spend the money patching them up once they're already ill.

There's evidence for that argument in a practice like this where we have large numbers of patients who've had reasonably comfortable lives in terms of good diet, education, housing and employment, living well into their 80s and 90s. What that means from this practice's point of view is that although many patients do run into expensive wear and tear problems as they get older, on the other hand they do remain fitter for longer and that's really what we're trying to achieve. It's all about quality of life really and how we can best use the available resource to achieve that for the greatest number of people: our difficulty, philosophically, is therefore whether we should be arguing for more resource for ourselves or encouraging the Government to invest more in education, housing and employment instead. I think it's slowly dawning on some people within medicine that this is a real issue: one of the things that has become increasingly clear is that none of us is living in isolation and that if we really want to try and change things we shouldn't simply do more of the same.

What general practice is going to be like in ten, fifteen, twenty years' time is a key question. The increasing expectation of the public to see a specialist, get a second opinion, is overloading the hospital system, with outpatient departments seeing 4–6% more people a year, though they're not iller. As to the skills of doctors, there's an increasing recognition throughout medicine that if you want to be good at something you need to do quite a lot of it; the surgeons who do nothing but breast surgery, they're the ones to see if you've got a breast lump; it's also been shown that if you want surgery for cancer of the bowel, exactly the same applies; if you want thyroid surgery, it applies. As a male GP I do virtually no smears and see extremely little gynaecology, because patients usually elect to see a female doctor. Equally, it becomes a rarity for our female doctors to see a lump in a testicle, so they have little experience of that. We also have asthma nurses who are as proficient as most doctors. The point is that while doctors are all specialising and getting more knowledgeable about particular aspects of medicine, we still need the generalist, but maybe not a GP, who is relatively expensive. Maybe it's a matter of everyone – practice nurses, GPs and so on – using the skills they're developing and becoming available to three or four practices as a sort of visiting specialist. That way we'd end up with even more skills widely available, but without the high cost of their being based in a hospital.

Being based in the community releases a cost: you've got travelling time of course, but if you do a half-day here, a half-day there, you're transferring the organisational cost to the practice, and the patient still gets a better service. One of the ironies about fund-holding was that while it was originally supposed to foster competition, what it actually did was to get the fund-holding practices working together, sharing their experiences and learning from each other. The dialogue amongst GPs at present is the strongest it's ever been since the NHS started 50 years ago; we talk to other practices now in a way that we never did previously, and it's not been competitive at all, it's been a matter of helping and sharing and trying to come up with common solutions. We have actually, through fund-holding, been given the opportunity to bend the rules a bit, be a bit innovative – and we have a number of situations where either our patients are going to another surgery to see a specialist on eyes, or we have a specialist in skin diseases or urology coming here.

Patients often have a distorted perception of costs. When we originally went fund-holding, a lot of patients thought that I personally was becoming a private GP and that my partners were staying in the NHS. A lot of patients think, too, that if they're on a number of different tablets they're definitely expensive patients, whereas the drugs may cost pennies.

A common example, particularly with the elderly, is that they would be on Digoxin and Frusemide for their heart, for both of which 100 tablets would probably cost less than £1. And the reverse is also true. I've a patient with breast cancer who came in recently having heard about some treatment from the Bahamas which cost £10,000, and she was assuming that the reason this wasn't available under the NHS was cost. I asked her if she realised what the treatment she'd already had in terms of mastectomy and radiotherapy and chemotherapy had cost (something in excess of £24,000), and she had no idea. I was making the point that £10,000 for treatment actually isn't a lot: a bone marrow transplant for a child is £39,000; a liver transplant £50,000; the cost after a heart transplant may be £20,000 every year. There are a lot of treatments which are very expensive, but because patients have little idea of the cost, when they read of something being available but 'expensive' they imagine that the *cost* is the reason a patient may not have been allowed the treatment on the NHS.

That was the background to the Child B controversy a few years ago – all the emotion about the leukaemia and £70,000. For the medical decision-makers it was never the £70,000, it was always the question: 'Does the treatment work?' The cost was not the issue. I think it's one of the enormous strengths of the NHS that if a treatment is known to work the money is found from somewhere to actually make it happen. It's interesting that with patients who go privately to the United States for treatment, six, twelve, eighteen months later you often come across a small caption in the newspaper saying the patient has died. The perception the public has is very much of a cash-strapped NHS withholding treatment, but people have also got to realise it's naive to think that medicine, however sophisticated, can cure everything.

I think one of the difficulties we have is that the public perception of what the NHS is about isn't always terribly accurate and television programmes like Casualty and so on don't often help. People come to doctors with an image of heroics being achieved. If we were willing to be more frank with people and explain that the reason they can't have a certain treatment is that it will not necessarily change their life as they believe it will, then perhaps people might be more willing to accept it. It's politically very unpopular to tell patients they can't have something though (calling the process 'rationing' is very emotive) – and perhaps that's why Governments tend to steer clear of it, leaving us to pick up the pieces – which is certainly a source of stress!

People think you choose your practice, but the practice also chooses you. At the time I made my decision general practice was very popular and for every vacancy there were certainly 40+ applicants. Changed days: practices advertising now are pleased if they get two or three people to interview. Workload is undoubtedly part of the reason why people are moving away from GP jobs; we work considerably longer hours than most of our colleagues in other professions. And general practice remains incredibly intrusive into family life – the demands it makes are awesome.

People are, I think, becoming more aware of how stressful it is to be a GP: when trainees get a glimpse of what a GP's life is really like they begin to realise that in the past people really gave their lives to medicine. Young doctors coming through now are demanding a life outside: they want to come in to work at, say, 8.30 a.m. and go home at 6.00 p.m., putting in a 9½ or 10½ hour day like everybody else. It's a very different attitude. The difficulty, in terms of recruitment to general practice, is that maybe they're right, there should be a life outside medicine – it's quite nice to play with the children in the evening or go out or whatever instead of taking paperwork home and getting stuck in for another three hours!

On the other hand, we're immensely privileged. I know it sounds awfully strange, but one of the best as well as hardest bits of the job is terminal care. It's by far the most time-consuming aspect of GP work because it doesn't matter who's on call you end up giving the family your home phone number and they phone you round the clock or whatever. But the personal contact, the feeling that you're doing something useful in that situation, is the reward. And the team thing is important, the effort with the nurses and the people from the Hospice.

The hardest question for me at times is whether I would actually do general practice again. The answer is that I probably would, I just wouldn't like to see my children do it. I wouldn't dissuade them, but I'd hope they would do something else: end up with a better life. I like my job – I wouldn't work as hard as I do unless I did – and I think we've really achieved a lot over the years as a practice, but I certainly recognise that the demands on the family are pretty grim in terms of time and availability. It comes home to me in the things which I remember about my own parents – the difficulty being at a sports day for example, or doing things with the children in the evening – and now I see myself caught in the same way, and that's very sad. Life shouldn't be like that. Other professionals work hard too, but they have more control over the demands on them, over when and where they do their work. I think that's a big difference, even although sharing out-of-hours work has improved things. The worst thing for me has always been the call at 3.00 in the morning; I loathe getting out of my bed and I can never get back to sleep. You get up at 3, you go out and do the call, you come back, go back to bed, and from 4 to 7 you just lie awake. And then you've got to try and work the next day. That's the worst: I can cope with all the rest.

I'm not sorry I left surgery. General practice hasn't disappointed – in fact the satisfaction has exceeded my expectations. One of the bits you can never really describe is the reward of seeing children growing up. We had a young patient some years ago – a girl – with horrific eczema, and at the age of seven she would come in and just stand there, scratching the whole time. And I used to hold her hand to stop her scratching and talk to her, and think how disfiguring it all was. She's nineteen now, and a student; the eczema's settled and she's really attractive. And you look back at how this kid was, and it really is like the ugly duckling turning into a swan. It's wonderful. Things like that are the good bits, the reason why you'd never give it up.

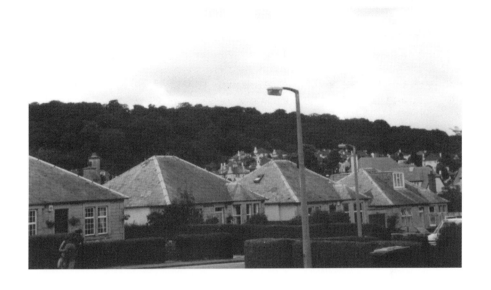

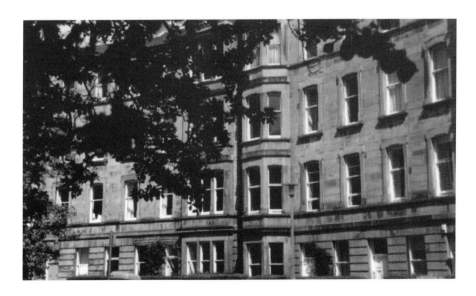

Neighbourhoods

3

Male GP
Graduated 1972
Location: Two-partner rural practice based in a small village

I was about twelve when I decided to do medicine. There had never been a doctor in my family and everyone seemed quite pleased with my idea, so it just developed from there. General practice wasn't a fashionable choice at the time, but once I got into my medical studies I very quickly felt that that was what I wanted to do, and my view did not change. I also had some idea of how and where I would like to work; I already knew this beautiful part of Scotland, and the thought of working and living out here rather than in the city was something I was so keen to pursue that while I was still a student I phoned up the local single-handed GP to ask about vacancies. He suggested I come and talk to him. As it turned out, he was moving towards retirement at the time, and to my surprise and pleasure he suggested that I go away and finish my studies and come back as his trainee, which I did in 1974. I became his partner a year later. Twenty-three years on, I'm still here.

My lack of interest in hospital medicine had a lot to do with how hierarchical hospitals were then; you couldn't be your own boss and had little self-determination. I was attracted both by the autonomy of general practice and by the kind of profile doctors had in rural areas; the kind of personal care they gave was something I very much wanted to be part of. And I had high ideals about the work I could do; I remember reading *The Longest Art* by Kenneth Lane, and being impressed by the argument that general practice is the hardest branch of medicine to do well because you have to have such protean knowledge and such wide knowledge at the same time. Many of the decisions you make on a day-to-day basis may seem quite small, but in terms of the lives of the people you look after, if you get them wrong, difficult situations can develop very quickly. In some ways of course, in a country practice, you are a bigger fish in a smaller pool, but you get back what you give. My predecessor was very highly thought of and very much part of the community. The idea of being, like him, a mentor and to a large extent a *friend* of my patients, greatly appealed to me.

The practice is now based in a single practice Health Centre where a female colleague and I currently share a list of just over 2,600 patients. From time to time we're assisted by a trainee. Consultations take place between here and a branch surgery in a nearby village. At the Health Centre we have two secretary/receptionists and a half-time practice nurse who, for the other 50% of her time, shares District Nurse/Midwife duties. District Nurses and Midwives around here are normally area- rather than practice-attached, so we're very pleased that in our case there is in fact partial continuity of nursing personnel between the practice and community services. Area-based Health Visitors also work in liaison with us. We have access to Community Physiotherapy nearby, but would like to see funding increased to allow this very useful service to function more effectively. Apart from Child Psychiatry we have no outreach Consultant clinics.

The socio-economic spectrum of the patient group here goes from an occasional class 1 through a predominance of classes 2 and 3 to some class 4 and very few class 5 – in other words there's a majority of professional, business and skilled people. Demographically half of the area is a dormitory suburb but the moor between the village where the surgery is and the loch is both a geographical and a social watershed. The much higher per capita income in some parts of our area is reflected in a higher level of car – or indeed two car – ownership. The social differences are also reflected in the use of services: there's an excellent local high school and very good feeder primaries, but there are also significant numbers of families seeking private education for their children, and about 20% of my referrals go to the private health care sector.

In general we have a healthy population: the considerable number of quite elderly people on our books reflects something of a deviation from the usual spectrum of disease: we see fewer strokes, less ischaemic heart disease, and less disease linked to social deprivation than many other practices. The number of elderly patients is a bit over the national average. While it's true that people do go on choosing to live in the area, it's also the case that many young people leave: there's very little indigenous industry so the young look elsewhere for work as well as for further education, and some also leave when they get married. Before the selling of council houses started there was virtually no private housing here that young people could aspire to, and it was, and still is, dead men's shoes for the housing still in public ownership.

A higher than usual proportion of elderly patients means that we do a lot more home visiting than is normal in many practices. Probably quite a number of these elderly people could come to us, but the home visit is traditional, and we think it worthwhile. I think my interest in sustaining the personal side of things through, for example, home visiting and open access to surgeries, springs from my belief in the old ethos, the notion of medicine as service. Marketeers would say that home visiting is old fashioned and that you don't get a clinical return for effort but to me it's part of just that personal style of medicine that I want to preserve. We're by no means old-fashioned in other ways; we're one of the top practices in Scotland for database development and other computer technology, and we have a very good up-to-date library. Our prescribing costs are 15% below the national average and we tend to prescribe generically. Once a month the six practices in the area meet for self-generated education, and we have recently joined up with two of them in a new system for handling night calls. In this venture we will, importantly, have access to each others' records. Innovations like this have to be built on co-operation and mutual trust, with the good of our patients always in mind.

In recent years there's been a lot of talk of patients' rights, of patients as consumers; the current focus on patient responsibilities to balance rights enshrined in Patient Charters, is, for me, important, as it would seem to indicate (and I hope it's true) that the consumerist pendulum has swung to its extreme and is now swinging back. I feel that the whole ethos of society has been undermined in the last twenty years because of all the emphasis on individual rights and everyone being out for him or her self. These attitudes have undoubtedly led, in some cases, to a lack of consideration among patients for the welfare of anyone other than their immediate family, and an unreasonable pressure on doctors; in my view patients as much as doctors have responsibilities to their community.

Getting patients to take responsibility for their own and their children's health is one of my aims, but there are quite a number of patients who are unwilling to do it. I do work away at it though. If someone comes into the surgery with a whole load of complaints and tries to off-load them on to me I find it a good technique to reflect back what they say, explore with them what they're telling me and try to get them to offer some suggestions as to what might be done about their problem. For example, if a patient of 56 who weighs 15 stones comes to me *again* to complain about arthritic knees my technique is to say, 'Well, let's analyse what we can do here. I don't think an X-ray will help because that will only show me the bones and we already know what the problem is. I don't think physiotherapy will help you much because you had that last year and it didn't do much good. However if you want to try that again – a few exercises, a bit of heat maybe

– we could think of that. As to surgery, if I had your knees, I wouldn't be letting a surgeon near them with a knife; an operation is unlikely to help anyway, but for someone weighing 15 stone it certainly won't! I think the hospital would agree with me there and would just prescribe weight reduction and paracetamol, so would there be any point in going? Now is there anything that could be done that you think I've missed? What do you think we should do?'

When you take patients through a situation in that way they begin to see how difficult it is for a doctor to get a solution to a problem without their assistance. And I encourage them to figure out what might be best. It's called patient involvement and it seems to me that it's respecting them as cerebrating individuals – better than simply grunting at them and sending them up to physiotherapy or giving them a bottle of pills.

I like to think there's some control to be had in terms of other patient demands too; I also try to educate my patients to judge when they need me, and they certainly don't call me out for trivial reasons – or if they do, they don't do it twice! I run a pretty tight ship and if patients abuse my goodwill, I usually tell them what I think. You hear stories of town practices where the patient who has asked for the house call at night for some trivial reason says, when their own doctor turns up, 'Oh, hello doctor. I didn't realise it was you on call or I wouldn't have phoned!' My weapon in this practice has always been that since we do our own night work they know they'll be answerable to the same guy next morning!

There are situations where you have to tread softly with patient responsibility though. It's probably true that in the past doctors abused patient trust in being less than honest at times; when I started in practice you didn't tell patients that they had a terminal illness; on the other hand, the American style of the time which was to say, 'You've got cancer, but we'll cure you!' was equally dishonest. Best practice is somewhere in the middle. In these situations though, you can usually sense when a patient wants you to take on a bit more for them, and sometimes we still tacitly agree to do that; I think that's fine – it's a question of negotiation.

Because of the higher socio-economic status and greater health awareness of much of our population there tend also to be different anxieties. I often remark that it's not a morning-after Pill people want here but a morning-after smear! We do also suffer of course from the content of the heavy newspapers, which leads to people coming in wanting their cholesterol checked and so on; but on the other hand the fact that people do read newspapers means that health promotion isn't a problem – the *Sunday Times* does it for us!

The influence of the media can be pernicious though. At the time of the last Pill scare there was a great stramash because the patients learned of it through the media before the doctors had been informed of the details. This, as I said in a letter to *The Times*, was both ridiculous and unnecessary because there is in existence a perfectly efficient system of ministerial embargo on information. Because of government committee work I often see copies of ministerial speeches three days before they're made, and so do the journalists, but in those situations they know that they would only get away with breaking the embargo once; thereafter the lobby correspondents simply wouldn't be given access to the information. The same conditions could easily be applied to these scare situations; an embargo would give time for the BMA, the Chief Medical Officer and doctors' representatives to prepare their response, and this would be infinitely preferable to the kind of scaremongering which ends up with people shouting down the phone at doctors who've only just heard the news themselves. It's awful when I'm driving home and I hear, for example, that a drug which I've been using happily for twenty years has now been banned. My heart sinks! The same was true of the MMR (Measles, Mumps, Rubella) immunisation scare. Because the media didn't put it over in a responsible way, the release of that information led to doctors spending whole mornings on the phone, trying to explain to understandably worried parents what the issues really were.

To be fair, though, the media, as I've mentioned already, can also be very good at handling health stories. Take, for example, the way in which they have publicised and promoted breast screening as the greatest thing since sliced bread; that has really encouraged women to go along and so, in their way, newspapers have helped save lives. But when, on the other hand, you get a bald headline saying: WOMEN DIE FROM MISREAD CANCER SCREENING AT X— HOSPITAL – that just sends unnecessarily wide ripples of fear through the population. The real problem doctors have to deal with as regards the media is that they have a double-edged interest in health issues, and the sensational headlines that accompany the reporting of 'health scandals' is primarily about selling newspapers. We're quite lucky here in that there's quite a reasonable level of education among our patients, but for those who are less able to take a step back and think that, despite what the paper says, they should keep calm, these episodes are very destructive.

I mentioned earlier that this is a training practice. I've always been very interested in medical education and became a trainer very young. At that time everyone was talking about the mechanics of medical education whereas now we look at educational theory and modify it for medical contexts. At an early stage I also became a representative on the local Medical committee and a year later was sent as the junior member to the Scottish General Medical Services Committee (the GP Committee in

Scotland). From there I became involved with the Rural Practice sub-committee in London and then with post-graduate training. Although a lot of my committee work focuses on having a working knowledge of the mechanics of it all so you can trade jargon with people, it's more the organisation of medical education and trying to raise its political profile so that it gets its fair share of NHS resources that drives me.

Being one of the moving forces that's trying to introduce summative assessment into GP training reflects my interest in professionalism. I believe that professionals should be self-determining and set their own standards subject to public scrutiny. That's also why I'm interested in the General Medical Council; I think that if we ever stop recognising the importance of continuing education, or if we hand over control of it to the NHS, we will cease to be a profession. The Post-Graduate Education allowance for GPs is just a government sleight of hand which involves taking away £2,000 a year from our salaries and then making us jump through educational hoops to get it back again. The government has also introduced artificial categories of 'educational' activity which don't fit medical education. Making doctors do things which, if we're blunt, have no real educational value is a somewhat tainted consequence of pharmaceutical industry involvement. Things like company lunches and so on are educationally very dubious. I think we should grasp the nettle and keep professional control ourselves, otherwise responsibility will pass to a Management Executive wanting things like Charters which include silly, anodyne expressions like, 'We will respect you (the patient) as a person'. If, for twenty-odd years, I've been working to the best of my ability as a general practitioner, what do they imagine I've been doing anyway?

The NHS is extremely important to our ethos as doctors because almost all of us believe that healthcare should be free to everyone at the point of use and should be publicly supported through taxation – indeed it's an irony that doctors, who tend to be very middle-class and conservative in terms of change, should generally subscribe to something that is essentially a socialist principle! The NHS is the last representation of the old-fashioned public service ethos, but they've now tried to graft on a business ethic, make a market out of it, and reduce patients to commodities; it all seems very inappropriate. From our point of view, the trouble with the NHS is that it's a monopoly employer and sometimes gets too much power. The medical profession is at least a hundred years older than the NHS and has been organised as a profession that long. What many people don't grasp is that it's simply the *method* of delivering medical care over the last fifty years that has been handed to the NHS as a structure: as I keep reminding their Chief Executive, if all the health administrators disappeared off the face of the earth tomorrow there would still be patients needing doctors. So I get upset when Health Boards talk about 'our (i.e. *their*) patients' because it gives completely the wrong impression; Health Boards are simply there to effect decisions we as doctors make about the care of *our* patients in *our* consulting rooms.

Another aspect of my interest in medical education is to do with quality assurance: I do actually think that practices should require accreditation and that professional re-accreditation of GPs should be tied to a mentored approach to personal educational needs and the fulfilling of roles. That's what we, as a profession, have to provide for ourselves. And we need carrots and sticks. If a certain sum of money were to be made available to *all* the partners of an accredited practice that would (importantly) empower the juniors. One of the great difficulties with group practices at present is that it only needs one or two older partners to be uninterested in change for a young, freshly-painted, eager-for-change trainee to run into the treacle of apathy or resistance. A trainee able to claim an equal share of funds could progress her or his ideas much better. Unfortunately this approach doesn't find favour politically at the moment, though things are changing...

There's a fairly wide spectrum in terms of quality in general practice though I'm glad to say that in Scotland at least I think it's narrowing with the weighting towards the good end. But there are still practices which do need to change. Training practices are different; they do have high standards; but only 10% of doctors and 25% of practices are involved at present, and naturally the training practices tend to liaise most with each other. We sometimes forget there are problems out there, that some people are drowning not waving! Those people need to be helped to change. One good thing is that the trainees themselves – young, good, idealistic doctors coming from quality practices where they have experienced high standards – act as an engine of quality which is to the benefit of both patients and medicine.

That kind of quality *is* the aim of the Management Executive of the NHS but so far they've gone about achieving it in a way that has taken away a lot of our self-determination. Doctors are understandably resentful as well as being exhausted by change. The morale in general practice is as low as I've ever seen it and it's reflected in an imminent and worsening crisis in recruitment and retention of general practitioners: firstly we have, at present, something like 20% of all training posts in Scotland lying empty and many doctors who used to dispute the suggestion they should retire at 70 are now eager to go at 55; secondly, around 75% of entrants to general practice are now women who may want career breaks for child-rearing or other family commitments; thirdly, an enormous number of inner-city doctors, many of them originally from third world countries, are set to retire; the problem is one of a serious draining away of people within the profession and inadequate numbers of new recruits to fill the gap.

So how do we move forward? It's been suggested that the whole skill mix of general practice will need to change and that nurses will have to start doing more of the things that doctors have done traditionally: I'm pretty sure nurses are not ready for that and I'm even more sure the public isn't. We need to confront the issue about the high cost of wastage – people leaving the profession a few years after graduation. Levels of remuneration are also a problem; the pay of doctors was never intended to become a marker for the rest of the public sector but that's what we've become, so every time there's a settlement for us it's negatively influenced by enormous concern about the level of settlement for 75,000 nurses whose demands will follow. What GPs need to do is to strike a bargain on the rate for a clearly defined job and then refuse to accept all the extra responsibilities which keep falling into our lap. One problem with recruitment to general practice that's clear to me is that if you're a medical graduate in your early 30s with your training complete, you're unlikely to commit yourself to a job involving partnership equity and so on which is virtually *for life*, if, alternatively, you can go and do 10 or 15 months of ophthalmology or anaesthetics and then move on to something else. The levels of stress involved in general practice (which people are increasingly aware of) are also, I think, a big discourager.

The worst thing about general practice is the unremitting nature of the work itself: you get one problem solved and there's another just round the corner. And then there's the climate of constant change; you have to be very resilient not to go under. General practice also demands a huge personal commitment of actual time: I've done one night in two or (if we have a trainee) one night in three on call for the last 22 years. Inevitably that interferes with marriages, with family life: you try to juggle your obligations and your relationships around the job, and then one day you suddenly wake up to the fact that your personal life is falling apart around you because the demands are too great; not just for you, but for your partner, your family, as well. That aspect of stress is demonstrated in increasing divorce rates, increasing problems of alcoholism, drug abuse and so on among GPs. Cases presented at Service Committee hearings reveal frightening levels of suicide, attempted suicide, mental illness – so much so that the BMA recently set up a GP counselling line which is now being heavily used.

So what's good about general practice? The variety and the autonomy are undoubtedly important, but there are also specific areas of work which are particularly rewarding; for me, the two extremes of life – birth and death – are where the greatest rewards lie. With pregnancy and birth you have at best a young fit woman as your patient, and you're introducing her to and guiding her through a new process within her body. And you're bringing a new life into the world, watching mother and child bonding and so on – it's a great thing. In a perverse way it's the same with terminal care in that you're helping your patients come to terms with what's happening to them, helping them through the difficult stages, controlling their pain, helping them die peacefully. And you're helping the family too. There can be enormous satisfaction in all of that. I often say to my patients and their families that just as the body prepares a woman physically and emotionally for childbirth, so the body actually prepares a person for death, too: we, as doctors, are there to assist that process. And I remind them that dying is as much a natural process as being born. I get very upset when my patients die, but I see terminal care as a very important part of being a family doctor. I used to have big disagreements with the hospice movement for seeming to imply that you could only have a good death in a hospice. My view has always been that their aim should be to make themselves redundant in the end in the sense that if they could pass on their considerable skills of pain management and so on to the wider community they could eventually shut their buildings down. It's the *knowledge* they have in hospices that's important, not the roof and the walls; they remain centres of excellence, but we should all be able to do what they do.

Terminal care almost seems to encapsulate what the whole business of general practice is about – total personal care, individual care and care of the family, whole-person medicine. For me, as the doctor, the caring is emotionally driven to some extent; I'm concerned, not just about their actual disease, but about my patients' pain, about whether they're worried, about whether they're depressed. It's about holding their hand, listening to their fears, asking them if there's anything they've forgotten to ask me: the whole bit. Rewarding is perhaps the wrong word for how it feels, but for me terminal care is the most complete expression of the idea of the generalist who has to look at everything. There are so many taboos surrounding death; a lot of people take death on board intellectually, but few recognise emotionally until they're perhaps in their 50s and 60s that the clock is ticking, the pace accelerating.

Many GPs would, I think, say that the gratitude of patients means a lot to them; I've just despatched an elderly woman with lung cancer who refused to go into the hospice or into hospital. Her family were not happy about the prospect of looking after her, but I managed to persuade them to go along with what she wanted. Fortunately she didn't last long and when she died I was able to say to them how well they had done, how respecting her wishes was the finest present they could have given her. To get a thank-you card from them the next day, to know that my effort to read their fears and anxieties and handle the situation to their satisfaction had been appreciated, made it all worthwhile.

Thinking back over the last twenty-odd years to how I envisaged the job when I started out, I would say that by and large, things have worked out for me. I don't think anyone does a job for that length of time without at times thinking that they've already seen perhaps 90% of what they're seeing now, but there's a great danger of arrogance in that kind of situation, and so it's good that every three or four years most of us experience a critical incident which is pretty humbling and reminds us that we don't know everything, that we're all still life-long students. And when you come to medical audit, critical incidents provide great learning opportunities. I've had one or two surprises over the years in terms of diagnosis; errors of judgement is too strong a term, but I can certainly think of things that, in retrospect, I would have handled differently.

Doctors are often thought to be distant, arrogant dragons at the gate; a lot of that comes from stories in newspapers which, if you look at them closely, are never actually about the writer's *own* doctor. In general, on public tests of opinion, doctors are rated pretty highly, but people's own GPs are rated very highly indeed. I think that reveals a sense of ownership by patients of their doctor – which I certainly feel to be true in a community like this – and so if a patient leaves to go to another doctor I do feel hurt, and equally if my patients get hurt or die I feel a tremendous personal sense of loss. My view on general practice hasn't changed despite all the difficulties; I'm still doing something I always wanted to do, but I now recognise that to do it to the very best of your ability you do give your life to it.

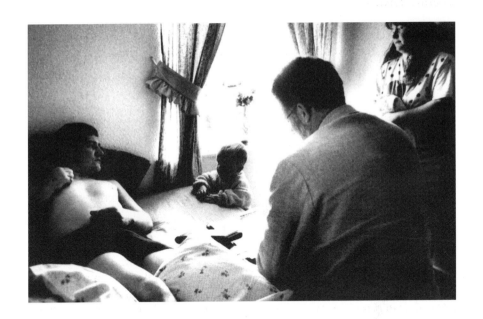

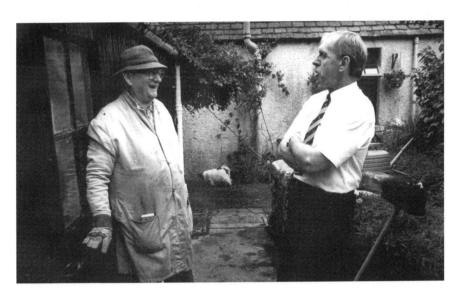

Home visiting

4

Female GP
Graduated 1983
Location: Single-handed island practice

I don't have a medical background at all: my family are mainly teachers and engineers. I did arts A-levels at school and was planning to do something like politics and economics at university, although I'd always been interested in psychology – people and so on. I'd also always liked our local GPs – a mother and son in rural practice who had always seemed very comfortable with the work. It wasn't until I got my A-level results that I discovered that I could still do medicine by going into a pre-med. year rather like people do here in Scotland. I was attracted by the idea of doing a vocational course and naively thought that my future might be easier to plan with a vocational subject. I was very disillusioned with school and I was worried that university might be more of the same but I went into the pre-med. class at Sheffield University and thoroughly enjoyed my first year; we were a very small group doing what was essentially a science-based course. And then I was dropped into second year where there were 150 of us, and I struggled on with this until I got extremely fed up. I took a year off and travelled in Africa, and that was really what made me decide to carry on with medicine. I worked in a couple of mission hospitals and saw a lot of health care going on and realised that because I didn't have any qualifications I wasn't a lot of use – I was really just an extra pair of hands.

When I went back to medicine my intention was to qualify and do something overseas. It became clear as I went through medical school that the best way to get good general experience was to act as if I was opting for general practice, so when I qualified I got on the Sheffield vocational training scheme and fortunately became very interested in general practice while I was doing that. Up to then I didn't have much insight into what it was going to be like, but I was fairly sure that I didn't want to work in a UK hospital, and I did become interested in the 'people' side of GP work. At the end of that six months I met C., my partner-to-be, now my husband, who had started GP training in Leeds for the same reason. We both intended to work overseas, but because we wanted to get placements together we actually found this more difficult to arrange than we'd expected. While we were still trying to organise it, two surgical jobs were advertised at the Islands District Hospital here. We were attracted to these posts but were advised to take only one of them otherwise we'd be working alternate shifts, and would never see each other! So C. took one of the jobs and I pottered about down south hoping to work something out; within a week of his arriving here however the local practice told him that they needed a six month locum and I then came up here to do that. When my six months were up I moved to another island practice and finished my qualification. I then did another locum job here but, in 1988, C. and I went off to Nepal. We both worked there for two years, by the end of which time I had a baby. C. then worked for Save the Children and I did part-time work with a mission hospital; I was really a leprosy doctor but I did some public health, disease control and so on. And then, out of the blue, I was contacted by one of the island GPs back here; the message was that he was looking for an Associate – was I interested in coming back? It was an attractive offer – people here had kept in touch with us very faithfully while we were in Nepal – so we discussed it and we decided that I would come back as the associate GP and that C. would follow me. I was then an Associate for four years; the Principal's job which I now have came up about 18 months ago.

We've been back here nearly six years now and have two more children. I'm the GP and my husband is now my Associate; I get funding to employ him for ten days a month. The practice is for the whole of the island; it's an inducement practice and we have around 850 patients. There are actually just under 1,000 people on the island but that includes a small RAF station. The service personnel are registered separately and my husband also works part-time as the camp Medical Officer. The wives and families are registered with me, though. We have two community nurse/midwives (one of whom is also a health visitor), three part-time receptionists and a practice nurse, and we're housed in quite nice newish premises built about six years ago.

The practice is developing fairly rapidly now. When I came nothing much had changed for some years. At that time there were only two part-time receptionists who also did the dispensing and we were generally short of staff. I've just recently managed to get funding for a part-time practice counsellor and we've started doing a lot more minor surgery and family planning work. For minor surgery patients used to have to go to the district hospital on the main island, or just ignore the problem.

I think on the whole this was really a 'curative' practice before, not much into health promotion. Women I think were particularly put off because there had never been a woman GP, and although the community midwife had made a valiant effort to encourage attendance for smears and so on, many women were reluctant to come. I would say that I've pushed all the preventative side.

The image and the function of the practice in the community has changed quite a lot; we've become much busier, but people still make some kind of judgement before they ask for an appointment. I do occasionally get called out for minor things, but that's fairly unusual. There are really two distinct populations here; the older island population, which is, on the whole, very stoical, and the migrant population of service families who are more used to a kind of dependency culture. I do see more of them.

The population mix of locals and younger 'immigrant' families is one of the things that attracted me to this practice. The practice I had been in before had a largely ageing population. I would have to admit that working long-term in that kind of setting – a small island practice where everyone was just getting older and older – didn't appeal to me. I particularly enjoy child health and so on here, and I feel that it's a very positive thing to have the service families around.

There must be quite number of low-income households here but people seem to be remarkably good at managing. There's a threat of redundancies at the moment because there's talk of closing the small island airport; that will be dreadful really because it'll be nine breadwinners losing their income with little hope of replacement jobs. And there's almost no chance of the women getting jobs instead – a lot of the RAF wives are bothered by that. We do have a leisure centre which has part-time jobs for women, and obviously there are shop jobs and a few civilian jobs at the camp and so on, but there's a lot of frustration. There's also quite a lot of stress which used to be more evident to the practice in a way because there was nowhere else to turn, but the RAF now provides a Welfare Assistant who's a qualified counsellor and she does a great job; in fact she's the person I've recruited to be our practice counsellor for the local population too.

Forces postings are usually for eighteen months; some people, particularly those with children, come and really like it. I think life here is hardest for the women who don't have a family with them. They can get involved in voluntary work but it's a very closed community – a bit of a goldfish bowl really, and everyone is so rank-conscious. There can be problems for the children too; some are quite unsettled from moving around. The constant moving also creates difficulties for me if a new patient has just started investigations or treatment elsewhere and I don't have their records.

I think a lot of the forces families do fear when they first arrive here that they've come to the back of beyond and won't get good treatment, but I'd like to think they quickly realise that for most things they're not really isolated. It's true however that the only access we normally have to specialists is when they come up from the mainland every two or three months. That can delay things, and we're not, of course, supposed to send out-patients to the mainland between times, but we do have a District General Hospital and a consultant psychiatrist and we're about to get a community paediatrician. There's probably an average demand for psychiatric services; the previous consultant psychiatrist set up a really good community mental health team but we do lack support for psychotherapy. It can be very difficult in a small enclosed community like this when it comes to people admitting to problems – particularly things like marital problems, sexual problems and so on. There's always the fear that somehow people will find out. It even affects patients' relationships with me, because although they trust my professional commitment to confidentiality, they do also see me all the time around the place – in the shops and so on – and coping with this dual identity can be quite difficult for them. It's potentially difficult for my friends here, too; if they had very personal problems they might not want to share them with me, but there's nobody else to go to. It's one of the problems of single-handed practice in a remote community anywhere that as the doctor you have two lives. This is why I'm glad about getting the part-time counsellor; she was slightly dubious about taking on the job because she also lives in the community and is very active in it. Dealing with the RAF families is different for her because they're so separate – but it will be interesting to see how the practice counselling goes. I feel that it will give people another option.

Counselling provision off the island would have its attractions but that's never going to be an option. There is a group on the main island with quite high-powered counselling training and that provides good back-up for anyone working in the field. Marriage guidance is also available on the main island, but it's not really an option to extend that service here. I would say that there are at least a few couples here who, if they'd had other options twenty or thirty years ago, wouldn't be together now. I think there are probably quite a lot of enduring marital problems in this community that are not even shared with the family, because the last thing anyone wants in such a small place is for relatives or other people to know that there are difficulties. Also, when people do split up here it can be very hard for everybody because the previous partners may still be around – to say nothing of the ex-in-laws! This can lead to chronic stress and some of that does come to the practice. Often it's a locum that gets people pouring out their problems because everyone knows that a locum's only here for a short while and therefore pretty anonymous. That may be useful to the patient but it's complicated in its own way for me, because I then need to be tipped off about the situation and watch to see whether people come back.

I don't think the range of illness I see here is generally all that different from anywhere else. We do have four insulin-dependent diabetics, all related, which is high for the size of population, and there are quite a lot of minor casualties because so many people are part-time crofters. There's also a lot of drinking and drink-related problems; the levels of habitual drinking which seem to be tolerated here wouldn't be tolerated elsewhere either physically or by the families. There's no particular age group or gender pattern to the drinking, but people are often aware that their problems are drink-related. There's a lot of resignation about drink too, so I don't really get people coming in wanting to sort it out or wanting a relation sorted out – they tend not to think that anyone could succeed! People sometimes phone up with harrowing symptoms but then say, 'Oh, likely it's just the drink, doctor!'; it can be quite difficult to persuade them to go into hospital or be followed up. I think that's the most noticeable aspect of practice here.

We also have quite a lot of cardio-vascular problems including hypertensives. It's taken a while to find and try to treat them. Hypertension probably runs in families but a lot of people do also smoke – and if there's real danger in having a high salt content to the diet then there's no doubt that having a lot of cured rather than fresh food – eating salt fish, bacon and so on – is a problem here. Having said all that, there's nothing that leaps out epidemiologically as being particularly significant.

My elderly patients are generally stoical to the last – many into their nineties and still living in their own homes. Most people are still looked after by a combination of family and neighbours, but we do have Meals on Wheels, and the district nurses are brilliant. We do regularly discuss things but they're pretty autonomous; it really is a team effort and I get to hear about things when they decide I need to. Visiting well, elderly patients regularly would be quite hard for me in terms of available time, though I know that some island GPs do this. I know of one GP who has an annual cycle of visiting, just looking out for problems arising.

I feel so lucky with the nurses; it is a lottery with new staff because I, as the doctor, have no say about who comes – they're just sent by the Health Board and one has to hope that new people will fit in. I'm not the nursing staff line manager either, though I can ask them very politely to do things. It's probably quite a good arrangement in its way.

Because of its unpredictable nature, terminal care is very complex and draining for a single-handed GP, and this again is where the team is so important. I really couldn't manage without them. Providing terminal care at home means that everyone has to be available round the clock, and this is physically and emotionally pretty taxing for me and for the nurses too. Even though they'd be entitled to, they wouldn't think of taking a holiday if we're involved in terminal care because they know that we would just have no one else to turn to. There's only one Macmillan Nurse for all the islands so she can't actually do any direct work with patients; she just advises. And our financial resources are not great; I have only recently managed to acquire a syringe pump for administering pain-relief.

Travelling about the island isn't a problem and it wouldn't be often that I'd spend half the day in the car. The furthest point I could drive to from to here would take about twenty minutes. We do sometimes have trouble getting people away to hospital though; the weather can create problems. We have an ambulance here but, in theory, no trained staff – just a bus driver who takes the patient down the island and across the ferry and then down the next island and across another ferry. At that point a District Hospital ambulance, staffed by paramedics, takes charge of the patient. The RAF ambulance and medics kindly provide a back-up service for serious emergencies. We do have access to Air Ambulance so I can also get patients either to the island hospital or to specialist hospital services on the mainland that way. What we choose to do depends partly on the state of the patient, partly on the state of the weather and also on the time of day – the ferries run from about 6.00 a.m. to about 10.00 p.m. and generally speaking if we need to move someone during that time it can be as quick by ferry as by Air Ambulance because of the time it takes to get hold of it. Our worry at the moment is that the ferry services are probably going to be cut dramatically and that's going to force us to use the Air Ambulance much more. That will make a big difference to how people see the business of going into hospital. Even for relatives visiting, it's going to be very much more difficult with fewer ferries; communities here are very dependent on them.

The whole maternity thing is also a bit of an issue on these islands because the policy is that all births should take place in hospital. Technically, our consultants on the mainland are in charge of maternity cases here and they don't feel happy about home confinements in this setting – and I would have to say that I don't either. But there are women, from time to time, who do want to be delivered at home: part of their reason for resisting a hospital delivery is that this commits them to going down to the district hospital a week before their due date to await the birth because nobody wants to risk having to transfer a woman to the hospital once she's in labour. There have been a number of home confinements on the islands in my time here; I haven't so far been involved in any but no doubt it will happen eventually!

As a family we're giving quite a lot of thought, at the moment, to what we should do about our future, because we have big accommodation problems in our present house. There used to be a doctor's house here, but by the time I came it had already been sold by the Health Board to the retiring GP, so we lived first of all in RAF married quarters. We're now in quite a small council house – which is very cramped with three children – and we're looking to build a house of our own somewhere. But hearing that the airport is closing, that the ferries are being cut, and that the RAF camp might also be under threat, we are beginning to ask ourselves whether we should be hanging on here and making a huge financial investment. A lot of things seem set to change; in particular, if the RAF camp goes, I'll lose the young families (which are an important part of my practice), the school will be much smaller, and the school budget will plummet! There are about 100 children in the school just now; it's a Junior High School which takes everyone up to fourth year secondary, and we're very pleased with that arrangement. When my son started at a smaller school on the neighbouring island he was in a primary 1, 2 and 3 composite class and was really lost; coming here has been the making of him, so we'd be very concerned if school provision were to contract.

Being a woman GP with children is inevitably a juggling act, but everything is further complicated by the fact that my husband is working both as my Associate GP and as RAF Medical Officer. Quite often, when I'm coming home from the practice, he may be going out to do his work. We don't have child care at the weekends, but during the week we have a friend's daughter who's interested in having a career in child care living with us and helping out. She stays with us Monday to Friday and that's been a great help; just knowing that she's there means that we're no longer constantly looking at our watches and worrying about getting home in time to free the other parent to do whatever has to be done. She is more than worth her wages. Being on call is also a problem if you have no help because the parent that's on call can't be at home alone with the children in case they're called out. And just sharing work can be complicated too; I paid a locum to do the first five weeks of my maternity leave, but then C. did it for me. I think he would be reluctant to do it again though because it was very hard on him. I felt quite guilty about it.

One good thing, though, about living and working in this community is that everyone is aware of us as people with ordinary family lives and they are very thoughtful about calling us out. When I get called out at night to take blood from drunk drivers they're always very apologetic, and when I was pregnant they were particularly mortified to find themselves responsible for my being there at two or three in the morning. I think on the whole my patients here are considerate, and that's one of the things I'd be sorry to lose. I know there are doctors who have come here and left again fairly quickly because they haven't liked being so personally identified with the job and have wanted more anonymity, but I feel fairly comfortable with my role. I wouldn't have wanted to come here as a single woman though, partly because I think that, for all sorts of reasons including lack of choice, finding a partner could have been difficult – and it's probably true that being the doctor does set you apart a bit.

I think I would be a GP again – I certainly wouldn't want to work in hospital medicine. I do sometimes think I'd have liked to do more aid and development work overseas though; C. still does consultancies for the government – he's just come back from Africa where he's been looking at the feasibility of setting up mother and child health programmes – and there's a part of me that's dreadfully envious of that. But the career choice I made was made for lifestyle reasons in that I just didn't think that the life I'd have had working overseas was compatible with having children. What I do here, although it has its problems, is particularly compatible with having a young family because, while I am expected to be flexible and available to the patients, by the same token most of my own working day is fairly flexible. Technically speaking I work 24 hours a day, seven days a week, but the good thing is that much of that time I can be at home. And if I choose to have a break mid-morning to breast-feed the baby no one's going to say anything about it; that's wonderful really – I feel very privileged. When I speak to some of my women friends who are combining having children with working part-time in city practices, the total number of hours that they are obliged to be away from home just seems appalling. I feel very fortunate; the flexibility and the nature of my practice population, my patients, makes up for the inconvenience of being continually on call and, indeed, being fairly hard-up compared with the majority of GPs. Working in an inducement practice is financially complicated and in the early years it just doesn't pay at all. It takes a long time to catch up financially.

I think this place suits me now; I always feel when I come back from visiting my family in the south of England that it does feel like home, and I don't worry about being stuck on an island any more. I don't really miss urban pastimes. C. fumes about there being no cinema, but it doesn't bother me in the least. And I was never one to go to the theatre much; what I like most is reading and listening to music and that goes quite well with being fully occupied with my children. I do miss going to concerts but not enough to be prepared to accept working as a suburban GP in order to have access to them. What I miss most of all, really, is frequent contact with my family; they're so far away and it's so expensive for them to come up here. I miss them even more now that I have children myself. Having said all that we'll probably stay here for a while; although we do talk each year about the pros and cons of it all, at the moment there do seem to be more pros than cons.

5

Male GP
Graduated 1980
Location: Group practice in a deprived former mining area

I was born in Varanasi, a city of pilgrimage for Hindus, the youngest of a family of seven. When I was about nine we moved to Calcutta, and I eventually went to university there. Why did I do medicine? I think several seeds – some cultural, some personal – were sown when I was very young. Indians tend to believe a lot in horoscopes and religious men and so on, and I can vaguely remember that, when I was about seven or eight, a clairvoyant friend of my dad predicted that I would become a doctor. My dad was a very hard-working person who hadn't had much formal education himself, and I knew that if I were to do medicine it would give him great pleasure. There's quite a lot of cultural pressure in India to please your parents but I, in any case, was happy to do that: my dad always gave me a lot of support, and I had great respect for him.

Another cultural pressure in India is that if you're doing well at school it is *expected* that you'll become a doctor or an engineer. Doctors and engineers are both very highly thought of in India, and share the same high social and financial status. To be honest, I actually had a quite different dream for a while – to play cricket for India! However, when I qualified for university in 1971 I did apply to do medicine and was accepted.

Medical school was really a disaster for me: my education had been entirely in private schools which were British in style with high standards and strict discipline; medical school in Calcutta was completely without discipline, and I ended up feeling very bitter about my experience. I passed all my exams, but I never felt that I had done particularly well, and at the

55

time I graduated my self-esteem was really quite low. It also gradually became clear to me that to succeed as a doctor in India it really mattered who you knew, and I had no contacts, no other medical practitioners in my family. What was I to do next...?

As it happened, in the 1970s, professionals in India – especially doctors – very much looked to Britain for further study, and I began to realise that my future lay here. However, there were major restrictions on Indians leaving India, as well as on their entering Britain. There were also serious currency controls – so I had big problems. Fortunately, I had a sister living in Italy who offered to lend me the money I needed, and so in 1981 I left India with the regulation 200 rupees (about £11.80) that you were allowed to take out – and came to Britain. My plan was to do obstetrics and gynaecology – a sentimental choice: before I was born my mum had nearly died from a septic abortion, so I felt that she and I owed our lives to a good gynaecologist.

I came first of all to friends in Lancashire, but had to come up to Edinburgh to take the exam for foreign medical graduates. I had a few anxieties about taking exams here because my self-image was rather poor, but I also knew that I wanted to succeed. As fate would have it, in Edinburgh I met a friend from medical school in Calcutta who was already working in Scotland, and he asked me to keep in touch. When I heard that I'd passed the exam I phoned him, and he then suggested I come and do my training in Scotland alongside him. This seemed fine, and I accepted the invitation, but it was six months in the future, and meantime I needed some work, so I did locums. Rather to my surprise, the medical staff I worked with seemed to think I was OK, and I was offered a Senior House Officer job in medicine for two years – a very coveted post. Part of me wanted to take it, but in the end, because I had already committed myself to coming to train in obstetrics in Scotland and had accepted a post, I did that instead. As I got more into obstetrics, however, I hated it – not the work, but the politics, the backbiting, the whole atmosphere. I think, looking back, I disliked the atmosphere of competition, but it was also partly that obstetrics is a very pressured field; there are great responsibilities, and the midwives and doctors are very intense about their work.

I began to think I'd made a mistake choosing obstetrics, and went back home to India to think about it all. And it was while I was there that someone suggested that I should think of doing general practice. I'd never considered being a GP up to then, but when I thought it through, it did seem quite appealing, though I realised that if I did go into general practice I'd have to start training all over again. Well, that's what I did; I came back to Scotland, re-qualified, and then decided that I'd do the whole three years' GP training. I could have taken a shorter programme which took account of previous experience, but I chose this long route because I thought it was important for a GP to know how local people tended to feel about things, how they reacted to different situations and so on. I wanted to learn as much as I could. Along with other specialities, I found psychiatry very worthwhile because it also helped my understanding of the local culture; the same was true of paediatrics. Looking back, I think it was a great decision to do my training this way, because by the time I finished I really felt at home in Scotland. Eventually I was offered the job I have now, and I felt pretty privileged; it was a hard time for finding jobs and I was a foreign graduate.

There are just under 8,000 patients and five doctors in our practice now. It's a high demand, low socio-economic area – an old coalfield. At one time whole villages round here worked in coalmining, so now there's a very high level of unemployment – around 20%. We know that illness is more common where there is no work or no money, and we also know, in areas like this, to expect a higher incidence of social problems and psychosomatic conditions caused by social or mental pressure. Among our practice population we have a high degree of drug abuse, the main user group being teenagers. With the older people the big problem is alcohol, and there's also quite a number of women who are addicted to benzodiazepines. I personally don't deal with drug abuse; we have a partner who's really interested and he takes the lead. But I do know that at times it's quite difficult to treat these patient groups, because the addictions are just symptoms of much bigger problems; what people really need is a change of environment, a better life.

Our total consultation last year was just around 40,000 appointments – about five times the population – though in the past few years we've managed to cut down on actual house visits. Most of our patients are high users of the practice and quite a number of consultations are in a sense unnecessary, but a lot of the use arises from the fact that we're often the only people that our patients can come to with their problems.

So much of general practice is dealing with the patient's hidden problems, but people do also take ill, so as their GP you're always afraid that you might miss something important; you may feel pretty sure there's nothing seriously wrong, but the patient does keep coming back. We call these patients 'heart-sinks' – they're demanding, consult again and again, float from doctor to doctor. Sometimes, they just seem to want to be ill; their complaints will be focused on vague things and it's difficult to know what exactly they're wanting to happen. The problem is that when you're dealing with a patient like this who turns up very frequently (say they come complaining of abdominal pain and you've referred them on and there's apparently nothing amiss), you become refractory – and that's dangerous because they *could* actually be developing an illness and you might not notice.

I think this kind of situation affects many doctors: I really worry about it, and cope with it by developing strategies and understanding my own reactions, and trying to have an optimistic outlook. Some doctors cope by de-personalising their patients, but I don't like that because at the end of the day I feel we're here to provide a service, and we do get quite well rewarded. OK we're not superhuman, and these situations are frustrating, but we've chosen to become GPs and we should recognise that. Sure, the work is hard and often not very rewarding but that's not the patients' fault.

GPs see a very low percentage of disease, though in one way all the patients who come to us are ill, or at least not functioning as well as they might. As far as responding to all these difficult, time-consuming situations is concerned, I sometimes think that coming from where I do I'm perhaps quite tolerant, quite patient. I'm very patient with our elderly patients because I have great respect for them. In my own culture age and wisdom are synonymous, and I still find it difficult that elderly people are viewed quite differently here.

Before I joined the practice the other partners had already discussed moving to better premises. Luckily, we were given a large piece of land very cheaply by a local landowner and moved from three cubby-holes to a spacious building where we still have room for expansion. We knew what we needed – more space, computers, a new system for our records, a library, our health visitors and nurses in the same building as ourselves and so on. We were very fortunate in that the 1990 White Paper laid down guidelines and criteria for general practice, though I do think that the way the reforms were actually carried through was very unfair and created a lot of stress. For example, over about two years our workload increased by around 40% with no increase in manpower. That's frustrating, because you know when you're under that kind of pressure that most of the work you do is not producing results. When we had the Health Promotion checks it was a total shambles. Patient education is great in theory, but in practice it's quite difficult, especially in an area like this.

Since I've been in the practice we've done a number of new things. My special interest is diabetes, but when I came we didn't have a baby clinic, so I started one, and it was very well received. Having done paediatrics I was keen anyway, but the other side of it is that I don't yet have children myself, so I enjoy baby clinics very much. I just sometimes wonder whether I've maybe done them long enough. I also like doing gynaecology, so my training hasn't, in fact, been wasted. Just as much as all these things, though, I really enjoy seeing the grannies and grandpas; the oldest granny

I see is over 90. It's known within the practice that I'm the one they come to; apparently it's because I'm good at listening to them! I like to look after them well, though, so if I hear there's a problem, I'll do a home visit and then go back and see them until they're on their feet again.

I'm in the Rotary, and I've recently taken up two community projects connected with child abuse and family violence. These kinds of issues really concern me. At the baby clinic I see quite a lot of very young mothers – fifteen or sixteen years old. Many of them are nice girls, but I do sometimes wonder what they have to offer the child, who is quite often being brought up in a fairly poor environment. Having said that, I realise that when people here talk about deprivation I may sometimes come over as a bit laid back, but that's because, honestly, deprivation here is nothing to where I come from. A lot of poorer people here could help themselves a bit more with the support that's available: people in India really don't get a chance at all.

There are certain similarities in traditional family roles here and in India. Granny, for example, is still an important figure in Indian families, and that used to be the case here too. Unfortunately, in terms of support for parents around here, granny is definitely missing these days – probably out working, or still with quite a young family of her own. Traditionally, Scottish grannies knew all about children – how to deal with minor illnesses, what treatment, what food to give them and so on. The lack of a granny to give advice and help rebounds on the GP and the health visitor; we now have to take on all those responsibilities that she used to shoulder.

How are we to deal with this extra burden? When I started the baby clinic I made little handouts on how to cope with minor illnesses and gave them to parents; that on its own cut down a lot on patient contact – I think every mum in our area must now have Calpol or Disprol handy. You wouldn't believe it but when I was first here we'd actually be called out to give Calpol to a child! At least that's stopped, so you could say we've had some educational influence on our patients.

My biggest interest away from the mainstream work of general practice is in complementary methods – sometimes called alternative medicine. I got interested in these treatments because not long after joining the practice I became aware of how many poisons we were using for purposes like pain control. While it was true that we were succeeding in suppressing symptoms or giving relief from them with the drugs, a lot of patients were developing side-effects (which become more marked as people get older), or indeed tolerance, in which case doses were having to be stepped up. Neither of these situations is desirable, so we decided to try to cut down on, in particular, non-steroidal anti-inflammatory drugs – Brufen and so on. These drugs have innumerable side-effects and can actually be lethal.

I kept on asking myself what the alternative was for a patient coming in with a lot of pain. What could we do instead? About this time I was introduced to acupuncture; I did a course and started practising. It was, in a way, a rebirth, because I had worked on a project in India where we used acupuncture for minor operations. Cynics will tell you its a placebo, but I firmly believe it works, and in some situations works extremely well. We can't yet explain how, but that's because it's beyond the scope of medical knowledge as it is at the moment, and the problem about trying to solve the mystery is that you can't do trials. Certain explanations have been put forward – for example, that when you put a needle in it causes local release of some painkilling substance and also stimulates the nerve endings. Other people think it's faith or longer consultation time that brings about the effect! One thing is clear though: the demand is huge. Even six years ago around 26% of people were actively seeking complementary methods, and that figure is now significantly higher.

I offer two acupuncture appointments a day and there are always about 40 patients lining up. I wouldn't give it to everybody; I need to assess cases first. If the patient is neurotic or the symptoms aren't genuine I wouldn't use it, but if the person is hard-working and medication is not proving effective, I'll try. Pain is a vicious circle, and chronic pain has a definite element of depression associated with it. Because of this, I need to do a psychological assessment as well. I would agree that the positive atmosphere surrounding the treatment does help, but the needles work as well. Several kinds of thing can be particularly successfully treated; a mildly humorous example concerns our health visitor, who tripped and was at first OK, but hobbling around in pain two days later. I'm not her GP, but I offered to help her. She agreed, and it worked!

Another example is a man over 70 who came in with a painful shoulder. He had been given painkillers and injections by one of the other partners, but nothing had really worked. Because I'm regarded as a practice resource and patients don't need to be registered with me, he then came to see me and I asked him if he'd like me to try acupuncture. Two sessions later he was fine. There are many similar stories; I have a female patient in her 70s who suffers from knee pain. She asked for acupuncture and I agreed to do it. She's never looked back, and now gets a few treatments every so often to keep her pain under control. Acupuncture is good for sports injuries or anything else that's acute, and there's scope, too, for using it for the pain of certain chronic conditions: it won't cure rheumatoid arthritis, but it does help with the stiffness. I don't use it on children however, or on addicts – because smoking, over-eating, alcoholism and other drug addictions are behavioural: acupuncture can work for the physical symptoms but it can't help the mind.

I'm also trained in homeopathy and practice that too: a lot of Indian medicine is homeopathic. Homeopathy works very well with children, and for pre-menstrual syndrome. The work with children provides some of the main evidence that homeopathy works: a child can't explain symptoms to us so we have to observe. The approach is very analytical. Homeopaths do a lot of pain analysis – the character and pattern of the pain and so on – called repertorising. Homeopathy won't work if there's a mechanical obstruction or structural damage, but for chronic problems it works well. And it does have a scientific basis; as with vaccinations, the basic theory is like for like. Homeopathy is different from herbalism: herbal remedies are not standardised – so you don't really know the dose you're getting – whereas homeopathy is very precise. As with acupuncture, why it works is not as yet well understood, though there's a suggestion that there might be an electromagnetic dimension to it. At the moment, homeopathy is the most highly subscribed post-graduate course for medics in Britain.

Aromatherapy I don't know much about, but what I do know is that the history of its use is also quite long, and some of the oils used do penetrate the skin. There are various reasons for the recent resurgence of interest in complementary methods – the global village, American influences and so on. I think complementary methods are here to stay – it's a relatively untapped field. And while the approaches are very time-consuming, the advantage is that you're not going to kill anybody. I find great satisfaction in using these methods because unlike so much general practice, you not only make a diagnosis, but are actively involved in treating the patient as well.

I'm very interested in medical education, and we're recognised as a training practice. I've had to think long and hard about this though, because, frankly, we weren't really prepared for the impact training status would have; we've had a few traumas, and two partners have left. I feel that we should be involved in training because we're a front-line practice in a deprived area. Quite often trainees go only to relatively prosperous areas and therefore don't experience the whole spectrum of practice: they may, nevertheless, end up in qualified posts in practices like this, so we do have a contribution to make – but the demands on us are high. For example, it's quite difficult for me, as a GP with a lot of commitments, to find time to do substantial reading. I think our practice does have the potential to train GPs but what I think I'd like to see in future is a scenario where a number of practices are attached to a training centre and the registrars work with various practices rather than one, and have a longer total training period. Experiencing variety is quite important when you're training – even doctors in the same practice can have very different approaches.

I enjoy my work. General practice is a science but it's also an art; a GP, in my view, has to have quite a skill mix – analytical skills, interpersonal skills and skills of reflection. I think medicine is, in itself, exciting, but what also excites me about general practice is the patient contact. I like people. I've experienced hospital medicine and there is the chance to meet people there, but not in the same way. And because of the way you're meeting people, general practice develops you as a person. When I was young I was very shy, but I realised I was, and I knew that if I was going to be a doctor I would need to work at communicating better. To be a good doctor, and particularly to be a good GP, you have to be a good communicator, to relate well to people. I'd like to think that I can do that.

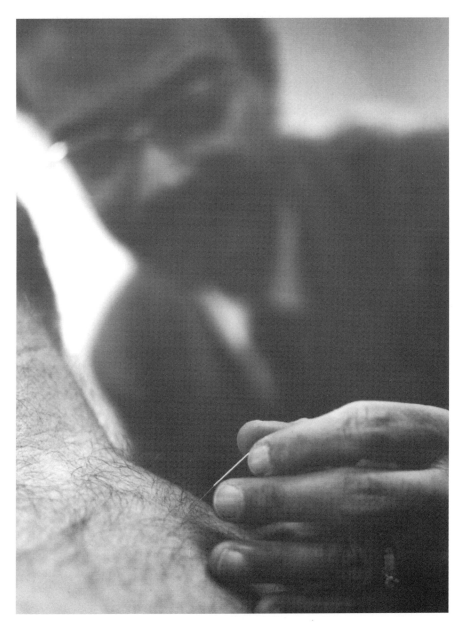

Acupuncture

6

Male
GP Graduated 1976
Location: City group practice in a mixed but largely middle-class area

My father was a GP, so I had a pretty good view of it all from close to. I think that when I was young I was instinctively more inclined to sciences than to the arts, but while there was the challenge of seeing whether I could cope with medicine educationally, there was also an awareness of just how interesting working as a doctor seemed to be. Medicine offers such variety that if you find your first choice isn't providing enough scope then there's plenty of other opportunities. Lastly, I suppose, I knew that a certain standard of living went with the job – you could more or less guarantee there would be no shortage of work.

The practice occupies quite a wide area from the city centre to outlying estates all readily accessible by car, and since we also have pretty good public transport patients tend to be happy to travel in to see us. Although over the years numbers of people have moved from the centre to the peripheral housing estates, many have retained an attachment to the city centre and to the practice. There's a sizeable elderly population in our particular area, but with younger GPs coming in a younger clientele has also developed, so that we now have, overall, a below-average proportion of elderly people, whereas when I joined it was above-average. We have big flats full of students, young couples – also in flats – moving up in the world or hoping to move up in the world, and many families living centrally and pleased to do so. Our patients have quite a variety of backgrounds: I would call it a complete social mix. I guess we have a preponderance of patients in socio-economic groups 1, 2, 3 and 4 as opposed to 3, 4 and 5, but I'm not exactly sure of the figures. Five percent of our patients attract a deprivation allowance of some sort.

There are three special features of our patient group: a significant Pakistani population, a young, upwardly mobile group, and a group with HIV and AIDS – usually combined with drug abuse.

The Pakistani population is housed predominantly in the large old flats; they buy these up and then one, or sometimes two, families occupy them. The men are mostly shopkeepers and the women – and the children too to some extent – help in the shop in some way or another, though a number of the children of these families have gone on to University. A bit of research done by one of our trainees highlighted, I think, a failure to address the needs of this group, particularly in terms of communicating with middle-aged women who don't have much English. Getting a female presence in the practice has, I think, been beneficial and meets a genuine need. I think I didn't want to acknowledge that for a long time, and I'm not entirely convinced that women always prefer to see a female doctor – I think they have, rather, an attachment to those who've been in the practice a long time. But I do think it's adding another element to the service we offer. I hope our female partner doesn't feel that she's getting only women's problems; I don't think she is.

The up-and-coming young with imposed or self-imposed pressures of drive, ambition and study and too many hours of work frequently suffer stress, so that their relationships are under pressure and so on. Helping them manage their health in terms of keeping the balance right is an interesting challenge that comes along quite regularly: I've always been interested in both physical and emotional needs, and I've acquired skills from my father and others that I can use to deal with their difficulties. For a while now we've also made use of counsellors, out-of-house at first, and more recently in-house. This has developed from attached counsellors-in-training coming on placement, but now we have nine hours a week of a qualified counsellor. That's a fund-holding development!

Dealing with HIV and AIDS combined with drug misuse represents a fairly heavy workload: the practice includes an area with the highest incidence of HIV infection in the UK. We've known about the problem for ten years now though, so there's been the opportunity to inform ourselves, to develop skills and to teach them to others. I've been involved for over eight years and it's been interesting: I don't think there's any doubt that the people of this part of Scotland have benefited from the way in which that particular epidemic has been tackled. At an individual level, managing HIV and AIDS is about communication and trust (if that doesn't sound inappropriate) between patient and doctor. HIV isn't actually such a big challenge now we have more knowledge, more skills, more practice with it; it's the drug-dependency that creates the biggest problems within general practice. Hassle at reception, for example, is something that has to be addressed.

Our practice team is unusual in that we're a group of three small practices – ourselves and two single-handed practitioners. The group originated in 1970 with three single-handed GPs, one being my father, moving into a surgery converted from a ground floor flat. They had two attached secretary/receptionists, and that was it. During the 1970s the attached nursing staff came along and the whole thing grew, so that now, apart from the doctors, there are two full-time attached health visitors, 1½ district nurses, three part-time practice nurses, a practice manager, a deputy practice manager and seven full or part-time secretaries/receptionists. Altogether it's getting on for 24 staff servicing the needs of 8,300 patients for primary care, so for this reason alone one needs some skills in team-building and leadership and management. If the Health Service is going to be led by primary care (and that's the stated intention), then there will *have* to be improved management within general practice. In many ways it makes sense not to have doctors as managers because they're expensive creatures and you can usually get a good manager for half the cost of the GP – so it makes sense to try and do it that way if at all possible. Also, if GPs are working quite long hours to earn well, then the management bit gets done at silly times of the evening and weekend and that then eats into spare time, family time. That's an issue we have to tackle: are we prepared to earn less well, and manage better?

The long hours in general practice, including time on-call, in the context of people's increased expectations of quality of life, *is* a source of stress for us. Over the years GPs and their families have looked for more time not tied to the job, and that's one reason why the drive towards out-of-hours centres and large co-operatives which reduce the individual amount of night work is moving at quite a pace at the moment. We'll have the opportunity to join just such a co-op soon and, strangely enough, probably won't until we see how it goes, the reason being that our out-of-hours is relatively light and we feel we offer a quality of service that is worth preserving. I personally would certainly want to go on doing out-of-hours work – it's simply another aspect of the job – and if, for example, you're doing terminal care at home, it's very difficult to do that properly if you opt out as you would in a co-op – though there isn't actually any reason why you couldn't do your bit as part of a co-op *and* give your home phone number to the family of the person who's dying. I've done that just recently to make myself more accessible.

Terminal care is first of all about choice – it's still an area where in a lot of places there *is* choice: here we have a day hospice and a residential hospice, the Macmillan Home Care service, a good community nursing service and GPs. I've no doubt that managing terminal care offers the broadest challenge of all to primary care teams in terms of teamwork, relationships, family care, working in people's homes and so on. Getting that right and anticipating problems as a team – all that is certainly where it's at in terms of satisfaction. I wouldn't want to give that up. I suppose a comparable situation in the past was domiciliary delivery – birth (to give it its proper name) at home – which I haven't been involved in, but which my father did for many years.

I cope with the stress of my job largely by taking exercise: I'm physically fit and I'm enjoying that. Spouses are undoubtedly part of the equation too: I feel that my wife listens to me, though she's not very tolerant of my deficiencies and she's right not to be. Certainly in terms of the effects of stress, the load on me over the years has meant that I'm not the husband and the father that I would like to be and I've had to look at that. When your family are reaching their teens you realise that unless you get on with it and cement the relationship you're not going to have one in years to come, so I'm having to be mindful of that. I haven't gone for any facilitation or counselling over the years, although I've had two periods where I would say I was mildly depressed. I've had one day off work in 18 years and have not needed any more, but I do take my holiday time when it comes along.

There's probably a cultural thing in medicine about not admitting that you're not coping, so there's a wish not to confide. You might think that since in our work we come to know people quite intimately we might be quite good at tackling our own problems, but I don't think we are. Our area recently instituted its own counselling scheme for stressed GPs, run by an agency: you phone a free number and they put you in touch with a local counsellor whom they engage. It's been used by eight or ten GPs since April and is actually open both to GPs and to their partners. My wife would like me to use it and I think I probably will because it's there; you can have six sessions with a counsellor in any twelve months. I would like to think of this as relationship-enhancing rather than 'repairing' – I could debate that with my wife – but we do have to admit that GPs put themselves and their relationships at risk through work. For me it's to do with perfectionism – checking things three times instead of once, resisting delegation to an extent. As a perfectionist I'm constantly disappointed by delegation; perhaps I should do more of it and it would improve!

GPs are not a homogenous group by any means: there's an immense range of skills. But there's a conflict to sort out, namely, what should be our core services? What can we be good at? What do we *need* to be good at? Do we become little specialists? Certainly for myself, broadening the range of skill and deepening it has been part of the interest over the years, so if last year I couldn't cauterise noses and this year I can, then that's a plus for my patients and I enjoy it. Similarly, if I feel that I need to become more competent in dealing with diabetes, then I'll do that – though the time taken does have to be weighed against whatever else the time could be used for. Given the range of skills available though, it would be good to let GPs follow their own interests through and refer patients to *each other* within, say, a group practice. We don't do anything like that – we don't sufficiently respect each other's skills; we tend to refer to outside specialists when we should be confident enough to take referrals on among ourselves. This is not, of course, something that would have happened in the more distant past, but fund-holding and the drive towards competition and self-promotion did encourage a bit of co-operation of that kind. At its basest, some would say, fund-holding was about keeping the lid on costs, right down to the primary care level. This meant that rationing became more obvious and more thought out on a day-to-day basis. Let's say, for example, that it was costing £45–£60 for an out-patient referral to a dermatologist; if I referred a patient to my knowledgeable partner instead it cost nothing except 10 minutes of time – though ten minutes of a doctor's time *is* a cost which has to be weighed-up. In a fund-holding practice, though, if the fund was not paying the £60 for the referral to hospital, then that money became available for meeting patients' needs in some other way – several hours of counselling a week, or whatever. However, while there are some decisions that should be considered at practice level – 4,000–8,000 patients – there are other decisions that I feel should be taken at the level of, say, 50,000–100,000 patients. I'm thinking of the situation where a GP doesn't see enough individuals with a particular problem to know whether the major rationing decisions about treatment should be taken. I only refer five patients a year to neurologists so how can I know what's appropriate? Equally, I might have only half a patient a year having coronary artery bypass grafting so I can't know what's the best rationing decision there: all I can do is to represent my patient's interest to the specialist and let him decide. There are many areas like this: another example – GPs who've specialised, let's say, in ear, nose and throat work in hospital, probably have, for ten to twenty years afterwards, greater awareness of the scope of that speciality than other GPs, so they may refer *more* for that reason, not because they're less competent but because they know the scope or they think they know the scope. It's only when the ENT surgeon turns round and says, 'Well actually, I've a feeling that these operations I've been doing on the nose for the last 10 years haven't actually achieved very much!' that you stop referring – which happened to us recently!

Another aspect of more overt rationing is prescribing costs. I had the experience six weeks ago of a patient coming back shortly after I prescribed for him accusing me of using him as a guinea pig because I had given him a new anti-depressant. He had talked afterwards to friends and looked up the books and decided that this was an anti-depressant that wasn't as much known about as some others, and he was unhappy about that. He believed that my decision to prescribe this drug was something to do with cost-cutting. We had an interesting consultation which ended with me compromising with him and giving him one of the same family of drugs, but one that had been around for longer. This is an example of how informed members of the public will challenge GPs – *Are you prescribing for me or are you prescribing for the budget?*

We can however compensate to some extent for prescribing expensive drugs by issuing private prescriptions for penicillin. A week's course of penicillin costs 25p, so a patient doesn't need to pay £5.80 prescription charge for a week's course: the chemist will charge the patient £1.75 for it, and the practice will save money. My feeling on the cost issue is that we have to bring individuals in – share the problem with them – be quite straightforward and frank, explore the situation if that's appropriate, and thus try and raise their level of awareness. I don't think we need to be paternalistic to patients; we should simply offer them our point of view and invite their trust.

There are many instances where we need to raise patients' level of awareness about the decisions that are being made. Our local health authority is presently debating whether it should in future have two maternity units in the city rather than one, the cost difference being about £2million year on year in revenue. My feeling is that we should offer the public that information, and also represent the alternative use of the £2million in terms that are meaningful to them – enough to buy so many more district nurses or whatever – because the population that wants two maternity units is a different population from the one that gets attention from district nurses, or the one that would like to have prescriptions for nicotine chewing-gum, or whatever. I think we need to try to offer people real choices and encourage them to participate in the decision-making. This may sound like a big change, doctors encouraging patients to take part in the debate about health care provision, but modern general practice teaching emphasises the sharing of decision-taking with the patient, and I see these discussions as part of that.

The future role of nurses in primary care is an area that concerns me. Many nurses, because of their instinct, or their self-selection, or maybe their training, are better than doctors in dealing with the less medical, more health-promotional aspects of primary care: the big issue for me is whether nurses should become the *first* point of contact. I feel that the drive towards that is financial: GPs are going to be asked to step back and become managers and planners and strategists and sub-specialists, and nurses are going to be asked to step in as the first point of contact instead. Certainly in terms of the clientele that we work with I would defend my role as first point of contact for a long, long time. Having said that, a lot of the development of health promotion has been rejected by GPs because they feel put upon – and probably because they feel that some of the science of health promotion is debatable – but when we look at the whole business of encouraging behaviour change – which nurses seem to be quite good at, and which GPs have not, I think, been good at – that's all to do with a sharing approach, with giving ownership of a problem and so on. If GPs can develop skills in that area it'll serve them well in health promotion and in rationing, and it will preserve and enhance relationships with patients.

Continuing medical education raises issues for me: how do we get GPs to change and to go on changing and forming themselves? Because of their self-employed status GPs can't be forced to change, but the development of medical prescribing advisors and facilitators has begun to channel people. To some extent it's leading from the front, identifying best practice and suggesting that it be followed, and to some extent it's looking at the worst and saying, 'Can we improve this? What are we going to aim at?' I believe that by and large we've got a pretty good standard of primary care in Scotland, so I wonder whether it's appropriate to say to already quite pressed GPs that they must improve. Shouldn't we be telling them instead that they're doing pretty well and will be supported in their personal development, rather than putting them under more pressure? There's the question, too, of *how* we can improve. The point was recently made by another GP that because we're used to short consultations it's quite difficult for us to adjust to discussing anything for longer – it's quite a lot to ask us to move out of that pace and style of interaction. That's why a team-building week-end away, having time to change pace, is so valuable to GPs. Or a whole day away at a symposium, or going into a library knowing that you've got two hours to yourself – different pace, different setting. We should do more of that.

I don't think there's any doubt that Trusts have sharpened up the way the hospitals' act in terms of seeking to meet the needs of patients and the needs that GPs perceive from their patients. The city here is just big enough to generate an element of competition in terms of provision. Professional managers have been brought into Trust hospitals and they've challenged the standard of all kinds of services being offered to clients, and demanded better. There has to be a financial downside of course, because you don't get new facilities around a hospital without spending money, and this puts pressure on clinical service budgets. We know the pressures GPs are under, but in hospitals one of the difficulties is that many consultants, as a consequence of serious under-funding, are now working 20–25% above their contracted time. My view of this is that they should turn round to management and give them one year's notice that they're going to revert to working 100% of contracted time and then *do* it for their own sakes and for the sake of the service. GPs might do it but it would be their own income that would suffer, so they probably won't, but both these situations of overwork reflect a serious problem within the NHS: unless the balance of funding is changed, I doubt whether the service will survive in its present form for much longer.

7

Female GP
Graduated 1983
Location: Inner city group practice

Why study medicine? It's the romance of it, I think. You see it as a good professional job which will give you great job satisfaction: you're going to do good and help people as well as being intellectually stimulated. I still believe it is, at best, like that. As to being a GP, after qualifying I didn't have any real idea of what to do, but I liked the concept of the doctor who knew the patient well: I enjoyed my GP attachments. Basically I saw GPs as giving continuing, total care, and liked the idea of being involved, being part of the family setting – the family doctor. Nothing else appealed to me as much.

We're a city and inner city practice, though there's a rural edge. All the partners in the practice are much the same age, so we tend to work fairly similarly. Because it's very much a young doctors' practice, we have a slightly lower than usual number of elderly patients. Conversely, we have a higher number of young fit adults and children, so we have a huge workload with things like ante-natal care, child screening, child immunisation, contraception. We have lots of big, needy families in deprived areas, and although deprivation affects our work, we try to educate people about how to use the practice, and the majority don't abuse the system. We encourage patients to come to the surgery if they can, and provide a lot of appointments so everyone is seen within 24 hours. We try to educate about treatment too: for example, we don't use antibiotics unless there's a good reason, and we explain this and patients come to understand it.

The smallest part of my work is dealing with patients who are physically ill and needing either treatment or investigation. The biggest part is probably seeing patients who need support in various forms which isn't available anywhere else – perhaps they don't have a friend or family to lean on. Patients may need support because they don't like their job, or they're unhappy in a relationship, or they don't earn enough money, or they've got poor housing – there are a lot of social aspects to it. To deal with many of these problems you have to have an immense knowledge of how to get things done (not just medical things!) and of what's available in the community. You need to know how to refer people on to other services.

A lot of my work, too, is involved in promoting health – in screening of the well, contraceptive care, ante-natal and post-natal care, asthma checks, diabetic checks. Then there's cholesterols, checking blood pressure, measuring height and weight, and asking smoking habits. Some of these checks may be useful, but a lot of them prove not to be. A lot of my time, too, is spent visiting patients: in a way this is a poor use of time because, despite our 'educational' efforts, the majority of visits arise from patient expectation rather than medical need. More patients living longer obviously generates more medical problems, but there are more social problems too. And more elderly people end up in nursing homes and residential homes that will call the doctor out to cover their own backs, so there's an increased demand there. Individual patients here keep their own doctor once they're in residential care, so when it's the flu season you'll visit a home and you'll meet eight of your GP colleagues also visiting because of the same upper respiratory infection! While I think it's nice for a patient who has had the same GP for 40 to 60 years to have continuing care, it's a total nonsense to call doctors out in that situation, because we're not going to do anything different from what the nursing staff of the home would do. Maybe we should think more about educating the carers!

The care of the very young and the elderly are significant parts of my work, and the nice part of looking after both these groups is providing continuing care. The young you really start looking after when you confirm the pregnancy and see the mum through her ante-natal care – and after the birth you visit the family regularly. We do child health screening and immunisation, so you see the children then and through any early illnesses – there's continuity and the feeling that you know them in the family setting. I find all of this very rewarding. It often takes time to establish a relationship with your patients – in some cases I'm still finding out about family members that I hadn't realised were connected – and sometimes knowing other people in the family enhances relationships.

With elderly patients, while the numbers in our practice are not large, they will often have been on your list for many years or even with a partner before you. They feel part of the establishment, and long-term that can be beneficial. It can be difficult for elderly patients if their doctor changes, and I think any new doctor coming in has to find their place. Particularly with the very elderly (70s and 80s upward) there's still the attitude from pre-NHS days that you didn't go to the doctor unless you were really ill. They were used, too, to old style single-handed practice. Most of the old folks have adapted, but some don't like group practices where you can't always have the same doctor, and some don't like the idea of a woman doctor!

Generally being a female doctor is an advantage, but there's a small number of elderly women who do *not* like it – particularly if you're young! It's different, perhaps, if you've worked with your husband, or been there since the ark, but we've had two or three elderly female patients who've made it quite clear that they haven't liked me and haven't wanted me caring for them. There's been no reason for it except that they've always had a male doctor. And while they can adjust to a younger male coming in because he's like a son, they don't like the idea of a young female. There's also a handful that would still prefer a male doctor to examine them. I think it's partly because they were brought up at a time when women didn't go into the professions – they would do something like nursing – and an elderly lady may not like what she sees as a flighty young girl coming in telling her what to do. You'd be acceptable as a nurse, but they can't see you *as a doctor*: there can be real disapproval. On the other hand, the ones I've had difficulties with have been so old that they've usually become a bit demented and then it doesn't matter.

With better housing, better nutrition and better medicine people are living longer but without the family support there used to be. Whereas before it was always thought that the elderly relative should be looked after within the family, that's gone now, and there's a huge developing social services structure instead. A lot of elderly people have difficulty accepting that as they get older they will begin to lose some of their capacities. They have an expectation that medicine can change this, whereas, while you can treat, say, cataracts, you can't do anything about diminished hearing or failing sight. I think people sometimes have difficulty accepting these problems and adapting to them, and they get very frustrated. Sometimes mental attitude changes as well, but quite often a patient has just always been an anxious person, and when they see their friends becoming unwell, passing on, they can become quite obsessive about their own health – and quite difficult, because there is nothing further that you, the doctor, can do. Some of these patients would have a better life if they accepted their problems. Having said that, a lot of elderly people are marvellous and accept ageing very graciously and with dignity, though even they, although they understand that they can't expect any more, may still get frustrated, and it can be difficult to keep the good will between you.

My experience of patients who are terminally ill, on the other hand, has been that they are very dignified and forbearing, though obviously people in pain get tired. No one has ever said to me that they would like to end their life, so I don't know how I would respond to that: I think I would sympathise though. From a practical viewpoint, if a terminally ill patient develops an infection (which they inevitably do) my own view is that you don't rush them into hospital, you keep them comfortable, and it's often a last event, so you're aiding nature to take its course. We all do that, but it's different from actively assisting someone to end their life. There's a crucial difference, too, between giving a painkilling injection designed to bring comfort and peace and one deliberately intended to kill someone.

With terminal care the big thing *is* taking time, and there's no doubt the more we're asked to do the less time we have for things that are so vital – like spending fifteen minutes with a terminally ill patient. Often the hardest part, even so, is working with the family, who put on brave faces but aren't coping at all well, and come and howl on your shoulder. It can be difficult after the death, too, as emotions are often running high and relatives may look for someone to blame. Very often, the GP or the primary care team are the first in line then. It's irrational and it's unfair but it's still very difficult to deal with.

Increasingly there's an expectation that medicine will prevent or cure everything. Because of this, when someone develops an incurable illness, relatives may think it's the hospital's or the GP's fault because the diagnosis wasn't made quickly enough: there's often a lack of understanding of the patient's situation. There's also, it must be said, the effect of the media's promulgating the idea that if almost any serious disease is caught early enough you'll be cured. I think a lot of media communication about medicine is good, but some is not so useful. It's frustrating if you've sat with a patient, talked through their condition and prescribed treatment and thought they've understood, to find them back two weeks later telling you that they've stopped taking the tablets because they've read an article or seen something on the TV (or their neighbour has gleaned something from the media!) which suggests the treatment is harmful or ineffective. Equally, there's an increasing tendency for patients to question what you're doing – and increasing awareness of what's available – so that some patients expect diagnosis and a cure immediately, and if they don't get that then you're at fault. I think the media can encourage unrealistic expectations, but there's also an increasing focus on patients 'rights'.

On the other hand, there *is* an issue of choice. I don't really think I'm there to say, 'You have high blood pressure so you *must* take these tablets…'

I feel that I'm there to say, 'Well, you've got high blood pressure and so...these tablets will keep you well–'. If the patient then says, 'I'm definitely not taking those!' then ultimately that's their choice – it's an informed decision. Prescribing HRT is another example of this: there's so much about it in the media that you must give patients the evidence for and against as best you know it and let them make the decision. In the past medicine was very paternalistic, and patients would often come away from a consultation not having understood what was happening. Now you're *almost* giving the patient a choice, though it still depends on the situation. If someone is really very ill and not in a position to make a wise decision people expect you to be more authoritative...

Care in the community is undoubtedly a source of pressure for the GP because that's the person carers think of getting in touch with when they need support. Communications between different parts of the official community care services are improving but more needs to be done. There's nothing more frustrating than doing a referral for a patient on the standard form (which is not a good form anyway) and never hearing anything more about the person, so that when the relatives are breathing down your neck you don't know what's going on. There's also an issue of inadequate resources for community care: at the moment, when you need to move things quickly in a crisis, the system doesn't work well. Discharged psychiatric patients, too, are very demanding of time, though often what the patient really needs is a *carer* – a community nurse or a therapist – rather than a doctor. That's a very difficult situation: often, the problem is not really about *medical* care. I do have hope, however, that GPs will be able to assert their views on these issues and get community care needs more sharply focused.

There is a general problem of *boundaries* in general practice: today many patients think that if there's something, *anything,* wrong you should go to your doctor. Working in an inner-city practice means that there's an increasing problem with drug addiction and alcohol abuse – problems that, in the past, were kept secret – but people also bring trivial physical things which they could easily deal with in other ways, and of course you get a lot of social problems too, partly because it's thought that if the doctor can't do something they'll know someone who can. It's so easy to get an appointment with your GP, and quite often, of course, we *do* know how to get something done. In a way we've encouraged the perception of ourselves as founts of all knowledge: the *Dear Doctor* columns in the papers tell readers to go and discuss so many kinds of problems with their GP!

One of the problems with general practice is that a lot of the workload is hidden from the public. People think GPs just do surgeries and visits: they'll look at the time spent on that and think we only work six hours a day! General practice these days requires an enormous range of skills: apart from the understanding of anatomy, physiology and health – of how the body works – and of basic pharmacology, all of which come from our formal medical training, there are other skills, too, like communication with patients, managing problems, which are essential. There are skills, too – like computing – that we didn't need some time ago. I qualified in 1983 and became a full principal in 1989. The new contract was introduced in 1990, so I've really no experience of the good old pre-contract days. The changes since 1990 have been phenomenal – a lot of extra paperwork, workload, business requirements, administration that you're not trained for. You stumble along, pick things up as you go, get yourself trained in your own time. The main training gaps for me have been knowledge and experience of running a business as employer and as *employee* of a Health Board, team work, team management, employment law, time management, managing difficult patients and difficult consultations, dealing with stress and abuse, dealing with government-generated goals – *changing* government generated goals! One law is introduced that says you will do *this* or you're in breach of contract, and then because it doesn't suit (because it's not financially viable) it's changed the next year. The classic example is health promotion guidelines which have been changed several times…

A lot of my time is taken up with running the practice: I do a minimum of two hours a day on notes, on prescribing, on patients phoning for advice, on having meetings with practice staff, educating, raising morale. We also have regular meetings with the Health Board, which have to take place out-of-hours. Then, if you want your practice to keep running well you have professional reading to do to keep you up-to-date.

Relying on the practice team as a support network is important and very much the way forward. It's vital to have goodwill within the team: if that doesn't exist it makes looking after patients very difficult. We have weekly team meetings to allow us to communicate with each other and with district nurses and health visitors. We also have people like counsellors and psychologists coming in, and as I'm the staff liaison doctor I have to spend time, too, with the Practice Manager. Obviously we have formal business to discuss, but sometimes it's just so she can have a moan – and likewise I'll have a moan to her! It helps to get frustrations out of your system!

If you're really finding your work stressful, help – in theory – is there, but in practice it's not. We have very poor supportive systems in medicine, all down to the assumption that doctors can cope – we're not human so we don't have human needs! Many GPs, for example, don't handle their own illnesses properly, as they would for a patient: instead, they'll go to their partners for ad hoc treatment. I'm very against that: we're all registered with independent practices. Needing psychological support is, in particular, seen as a sign of failure in a doctor, and we're poor at *giving* help to each other because of embarrassment and awkwardness about the whole issue. Personally I've been through an awful lot – big upheavals – so I know. We tend not to discuss our own stress in the practice and take it out at home instead. Stress and depression are well documented among GPs, along with alcoholism, drug abuse, divorce, even suicide, and until we're big enough to say we're human – that we have needs too – we're not going to change that.

We know that, for GPs, the stresses come from the out-of-hours commitment, increased workload, an increase in difficult patients. If the government would only support us we could definitely resolve a lot of the stress: if, on the other hand, our problems are ignored, there will soon be a recruitment crisis. Already people are either leaving the profession or not coming in, and those that are coming in are not taking principal status, so something urgently needs to be done. As a profession we need our leaders to be strong and they're starting to be so, but we need support from the government too, and they won't give it because it would increase costs, and it suits them that at the moment general practice is a very cheap service. If only we had a politician with insight who could see that we're digging a huge hole for the NHS to fall into – and because the service *is* so stretched and strained more and more things are ending up in the GP's lap. Every week you pick up the journals and read that GPs fail to do this, fail to do that, but there's a limit to what I can do well within a certain number of hours. We need the patients' support, too, because if we're tired, burnt-out, hacked-off GPs, we're not able to give patients the kind of service they need or deserve. The only way we could achieve that is by reaching some sort of compromise through looking realistically at what people should be able to expect from GPs.

When all's said and done it's definitely the patients that make going to work as a GP worthwhile: seeing so many different people and getting to know them is very rewarding. I think there's still a place for the more traditional helping or caring role which GPs filled in the days when there were few sophisticated treatments to offer: it's because we do care in that way that many of us have gone into general practice. And that's one of the things that our patients *do* appreciate too. One of the nicest compliments I ever had was from an elderly man who told me he liked coming to see me because I always made him laugh – it's a pity that time pressure makes it increasingly difficult for us to give that bit extra to our patients. I remember, too, visiting an old lady that we never see, who, though she didn't need to be in hospital, was quite unwell with sickness and diarrhoea.

On my visit I cleaned her up and changed her bed, and when I popped back to see her she was so grateful to me for having done these things for her. The days of getting presents are past – especially in the inner city – but you often get a thank-you, a card handed in, and it makes your whole week.

I find I have more self-doubt now than I had to start with; there's probably a certain amount of arrogance in many young doctors at the beginning. It's not unhealthy to have doubts but it does give you a harder time. And there are so many demands on your time that you feel that you can't give quality care. Complaints and the fear of complaints are the things that really get me down. A patient who complains about you or gets a relative to do it – that really hurts. As to the *fear* of complaints – we're much more defensive in our work these days: there's almost always a worry there that you've missed something, and the time pressure that we work under, and the range of work that is demanded of us, doesn't help this at all.

There are a lot of different views around as to how our problems could be resolved, but certainly, if we're to give quality care, it has to be recognised that we can't do *everything*: that just leads to inefficiency. Some people would say doctors are doing too many non-medical things, but while this is true, it will always be difficult to weed out what's inappropriate so long as patients are free to come to us with *anything*! The government has to stop sticking its head in the sand and address this issue.

8

Male (retired) GP
Graduated 1954
Location: Affluent suburban practice

Although I grew up in a village in Scotland, my father was French. He was from a peasant family, and because he had left school at the age of eight he was determined that I would have as much schooling as possible and go on to university. It didn't really matter what I did there, but I *had* to have a university education.

Why did I do medicine? I suppose our village doctor was the main influence. He was very tall and had enormous presence, and when he called, everything in the house stopped. I was rather in awe of him. Another influence probably came through a London GP's son, the same age as myself, who was evacuated to our village during the war. We became friends and went through secondary school together, and during that time I occasionally visited his family in London. Obviously I saw something of his father's life as a GP there too, and so when I got into my teens and hadn't a clue what I wanted to do at university, these two rather attractive images of family doctors probably encouraged me to drift into medicine. As a matter of fact, though, ten of our school year went on to do medicine – which maybe says something about breadth of imagination!

I made heavy weather of the initial years of medical school because I had no feeling for anatomy or physiology – in fact, till I got to about my fourth year I really wondered what I was doing there. It was only when I got into obstetrics, surgery and medicine that I began to feel that I had some slight flair, and by the time I qualified it was clear that obstetrics and gynaecology were the areas where I could shine, so that's where I headed. Having got my house jobs and National Service out of the way I began work in the maternity hospital – and I just revelled in that, even though we were working 20 hours out of 24. Before long the professor suggested to me that I might consider a career in obstetrics, but then another consultant who knew that I was about to get married told me to think very carefully about going down that road; we were all aware of how many registrars' marriages were under strain because of their having to live-in at the hospital with hardly any time at home. This conflicting advice left me in a bit of a dilemma, but then, just as I was mulling everything over, a GP in a very prosperous area of the city offered me a job as his assistant, and for what seemed at the time like good practical reasons, I accepted. I remained in the same practice for the whole of my working life, and retired seven years ago.

It was generally thought to be pure gold to land a job in a decent practice then, but even though I had made the choice freely, I was actually very unsettled for a long time, very regretful about not making a career in obstetrics and very unhappy about how the practice I was in was run. My senior partner had been trained before the war and had simply copied all the systems he'd come across in his own training practice in the north of England. The arrangements were excellent so far as they went, but there was no real analysis of the work, no imaginative innovations like ante-natal or immunisation sessions, no vision. And of course we had no *training*. Having got this straight Assistantship in a good area I was the envy of everyone, but the lack of training was a nightmare: I used to sit in the surgery sometimes and copy treatments out of the pharmaceutical books so that I wouldn't get caught out not knowing what drugs to give to patients. It was absolutely pathetic – and very stressful!

Added to my lack of experience or training was the fact that we had no secretary and no appointment system, so there was no way of reminding myself of a patient's history by pulling out records prior to their visit. In those days a GP was, in any case, supposed to *know* who each patient was; but while I've a good memory for faces I've a bad memory for names, and patients that I'd seen before would come in and I would be sitting there unable to concentrate on what they were telling me for much of the time because I was desperately trying to remember who they were.

In one way therefore the modern systems of general practice involving secretaries and so on have been, for me, a great development, but I do think things have been lost as well. Up until shortly before I qualified a lot of medical treatment had really been a kind of witch-doctoring. A few remedies *were* available, but by and large doctors used the power of their personalities to cure patients. The majority of people did recover of course – partly no doubt because a large proportion of the illness presented was self-limiting anyway and didn't need drugs. But then in the fifties doctors were bombarded with a whole range of new drugs, including antibiotics. The pressure to prescribe these new drugs was considerable, and suddenly we were using (and misusing) them on a grand scale – throwing penicillin, for example, at everything from the common cold to the most serious of pneumonias, and not really understanding what we were doing half the time. Looking back, I see that time as the moment when general practitioners began to move away from their old role of supporting people mainly through attention, care and concern, and started to become 'scientific'. In fact, much of the illness that GPs see these days continues to be self-limiting: it's largely because the patient's expectation now is to recover in two days rather than five that drugs are so much in demand.

I'm rather sad about the way general practice has gone because the old way had its strengths; now, especially in prosperous areas where people are well educated, well aware of health issues, we're having to practice medicine as patients expect it, and this is causing us to become extremely defensive and litigation-conscious. In a prosperous area you have to develop a partnership with your patients, respond to their questioning and so on. It does keep you on your toes however. By contrast, friends of mine who worked as GPs in poor areas would admit that because their patients rarely questioned them about diagnosis or prescribing their practice was, at times, in danger of becoming insufficiently self-critical or even lazy.

The range of things people present to GPs has increased enormously over the last forty years or so – there are many more psycho-social problems for example. In the late 1950s many of us had never, so far as we knew, seen a homosexual patient – but of course we weren't looking for them, and we had no psychiatric training that might have provided us with insights. Although training is now provided, I think many GPs still find it difficult to deal with some of these very sensitive areas of casework – indeed with anything of an emotional nature that they haven't come to terms with personally. Doctors are no different from the rest of the population, and just as there are patients who never accept that they're unwell or that their family are unwell and are therefore pretty unsympathetic if, say, their wife is suffering from depression, so GPs are tuned in to different things. My patients used to tell me that the most important thing I gave them was the sense that (mostly) everything would be all right – and it usually was! That was probably a case of my practice reflecting my own reasonably optimistic view of life, but once I became aware of this dynamic my whole interest in practice eventually focused on how, through my interaction with them, I *could* affect my patients' outlook and attitudes to life. It was great to be able to so subtly stimulate patients to self-help that they thought they had made decisions themselves. In the old days GPs were very directive, but gradually they've learnt to sit and listen more and simply give encouraging signs. Some would say that today the 'scientific' role of the general practitioner – factual diagnosis, positive treatment and so on – is paramount, and the doctor/patient relationship is less important, but when I retired I realised that what I valued most and what I missed was not the medicine but the interaction with people. That, for me, is *the* function of the general practitioner.

The modest practice I started in grew, in thirty years, from just one full-time GP, a part-timer (his wife) and an assistant (myself) serving under 3,000 patients, to a group practice of five doctors serving between 10,000 and 11,000 patients. The introduction of practice nurses, health visitors, counsellors and so on has unquestionably diminished the general practitioner's sphere of influence. I, for instance, right up to retiral, continued to visit my 'chronics' personally. Critics would say that this can equally well be done by nursing staff, and that doctors only do it because of the good feelings they get from helping people who admire them and so on; well, there might be a bit of that, but it's not the whole story. When I retired I was still seeing chronically ill patients not much older than myself that I had been looking after ever since we were all young. Of course these patients become very dependent on you, but they also become friends. They're very easy to treat therefore: even if one danger in seeing people often is that you may miss an obvious diagnosis, the advantage is that when you know people so well you can see a crisis coming. And as such patients age within their own homes, you see new difficulties arise and can anticipate the different kinds of help that will be required. I was always being accused by my younger partners of stirring up older patients to think that they weren't going to manage so well at home in future – that I was living their lives for them (and sometimes they may have been right!) but I was usually simply anticipating real problems and getting them aired. Because of regular visiting I could see someone becoming unfit to manage the house with stairs and outside coal sheds and so on. Now in one way these *are* lay matters rather than medical problems, and it could be argued that they should be dealt with by someone other than a GP; I would contend however that they are appropriate areas of concern for a GP to become involved in as part of whole-person medicine. It's only because we're living at a time when concepts of value in the health service are being constantly reduced to issues of economics that the time spent by a GP in dealing with such personal problems is seen as unjustifiable.

Home visits in general have suffered from the hard economic approach; that's regrettable in some ways because home visits can be so revealing, so valuable to the GP trying to appreciate the patient's situation. As soon as you enter a house you see reflections of the family's or the individual's life, and if you're receptive enough to these you might be asking yourself whether there's any kind of situation there – emotions, relationships – that might be contributing to, for example, a wife's depression or a kid's constant asthmatic attacks. The cost-conscious however would again argue that this kind of attention to 'non-medical' detail is an inappropriate use of a doctor's costly time and belongs in a deluxe health service which we simply can't afford. My response to that would be to ask whether many of the tasks that we currently consider it *appropriate* for GPs to perform are an effective use of funds or whether present arrangements actually prevent most doctors from reaching their ceiling of ability and exercising their highest levels of skill. For years I've believed much of the routine work of general practice to be quite within the competence of a properly but much less expensively trained person; a new breed of auxiliary GPs – such as you find in Germany – or even advanced nurse practitioners could be trained to pick up on key symptoms, treat the simpler more straightforward ailments themselves, and refer on the more complex cases. I have no problem with this because I can recall that when my generation came out of medical school our ideas about disease and our practical skills were very basic. I don't remember ever being able to see an ear drum before I came into general practice; I had to learn on the job. I never looked at a sore throat before I got into practice – so I learnt that on the job too. I therefore don't accept that it needs a full medical school training to acquire the necessary level of skill for a job where the same recurrent illnesses make up the bulk of the workload. If we adopted this approach we could also have a more cost-effective structure to primary care. Doctors, as a profession, are not supposed to say that of course as it's not in our own interest to imply that society doesn't really need so many of us!

In my view the health service has recently spent too much money paying doctors to do things which are either not sufficiently complex to justify the cost of their training, or not directly to do with looking after people at all. Take fund-holding for example; why were expensively trained doctors offered incentives to learn how to do financial jobs which could be better done by people with an accountancy background? A cynical explanation might be that individually and collectively we recognise that the boredom factor in general practice is quite high, and so it's a very attractive proposition for the average GP to go off and do something else for a change. I have no doubt that when I worked for the Industrial Medical Board or started teaching for the local University Department of General Practice I was trying to get out of general practice, to find an alternative which would keep me sane and allow me to go back to the surgery and yet again see Mrs Smith with her dozen complaints which I knew I couldn't resolve.

When I was a young GP the work really interfered with family life; we worked each day till the work was finished and then did large amounts of out-of-hours duty. Surgeries ran on endlessly because if someone came in with six complaints I felt bound to honour all six whether I could actually do something about each one or not. Recently trained GPs work differently; a young GP now will offer to deal with one or two complaints meantime, ask the patient to come back about the others at some future date, and worry less. That's training, and patients generally accept how their GP works – or they go elsewhere. When a GP is in practice in one place for any length of time the patients get a fairly clear sense of how he feels about their visits. If the doctor's approach is welcoming however trivial the problem, if he treats patients well and makes them feel that their visit is justified, they'll feel free to come back often. The problem here is that word gets around that this doctor is approachable, and the number of patients coming along with trivial complaints that they feel the other partners have no time for will increase. It's important to remember of course that there's not only the patient in this interaction, there's the doctor as well. It might be in his own interests to get trivial cases to come back – the workload then is much easier, the pressure is much less; and there's little space for new patients – new patients meaning 'new problems' requiring thinking, action, decisions, demanding greater effort! If a doctor wants an easy life, then a regular supply of well-known faces with nothing very seriously wrong with them can be a very attractive arrangement.

I've touched already on the repetitive nature of the work and lack of challenge that GPs can experience. To help counteract this there's a need, I think, to provide greater structure to their careers. For a start, it's quite wrong to bring young doctors into a practice and have them, within a couple of years, on parity with everybody else. My reason for saying this is not that I think younger doctors should be less well paid; it's rather that I feel it's bad psychologically for a young professional to be able to reach their peak of achievement so soon when they have another 30 years or so to work. General practice is very different from hospital medicine in this respect; it would be better for people to come into practice at a junior level and work up through various stages over a longer time scale, acquiring full responsibility, participation in planning and so on more gradually. There is a drawback here, however, in that some of the young people in general practice are the very ones with the good ideas, and a more rigid career structure could hold such people back; but on the other hand I would hope that a sound structure and good management would allow even a very young person to contribute without damping down enthusiasm.

General practice could also provide an excellent opportunity for a career break; one could work as a GP up to, say, 40 or 45 and then go on to something else. The repetitive nature of much general practice means that it becomes very stultifying to someone with a good intellect. An ideal society would have another sphere of public service into which interested and able GPs could go and contribute their expertise to dealing with the needs of families, the structuring of preventive care and so on. Some practices used fund-holding to allow individuals to pursue their own interests and develop expertise which would be of general use. The thought of using each other as experts is not new, but there are practicalities to be sorted out – for example people have to agree to being used like this and decide among themselves who will be the paediatric specialist, the psychiatric specialist and so on, and time used in these specialist ways has to be balanced with everyone else's time spent doing the routine jobs. One problem of course is that the longer you are in general practice – unless you keep in touch with a specialist department – the more danger there is of your view becoming dated, and not necessarily better than that of a recent registrar. In that situation, why should people turn to you as the expert?

General practice has to some extent lost its way. Traditionally, the general practitioner was a father figure in the community who fulfilled a host of roles, but, in particular, cared in a most personal way for his patients. In the past it was recognised that a good GP needed to possess a wide range of skills, not all of them measurable by academic examinations; but because of the way in which medicine has become more 'scientific', we now feel the need to recruit the brightest to medical schools and give them an essentially science-based training.

Criteria for recruiting medical students need to be re-examined in my view; when I sat on a University Admissions Committee, one of the things which astounded and depressed me was the way in which it was deemed appropriate to go chasing after the top A level students from England before Oxford or Cambridge got them. I have never understood why high entrance qualifications should be thought necessary for medicine: medical training is actually quite narrow and in many ways not particularly demanding intellectually. Students progress, in the main, by learning up facts and spewing them back, and pass their exams on the basis of learning up diagnosis and treatment. There's little scope for originality!

We must also think harder about what we're ultimately going to use such high flying recruits for. Of course there are research areas in medicine for which one does need a first class analytical mind and a capacity for great breadth of knowledge and understanding, but I don't believe that the average physician or surgeon needs to be in that league, and general practitioners certainly don't. What general practitioners need is a very sound average brain coupled with a sense of dedication and the ability and temperament to cope with repetitive work. For all the recent emphasis on 'scientific' training, medical graduates who progress to general practice soon discover, just as they did in my day, that a GP's job involves dealing not just with strictly medical problems but with a thousand and one other things which 'scientific' training has ill-equipped them for.

I suspect that what underlies much of the fuss about entrance qualifications for medical school is something of the myth of the doctor, which is deep in our culture: because we invest them with such trust and status we cannot allow doctors to be just average people – but why? During my time in general practice roughly 20–30 trainees worked with us, starting, in the early years, with pretty averagely qualified students, and ending with high fliers. I could never say hand on heart that I recognised any difference between the average people and those who were supposed to be very bright. They certainly didn't make better doctors.

My heart is obviously with the traditional role of the GP, but even I recognise that the day of that personal kind of medicine is probably over and that the 'scientific' approach to general practice is here to stay. The question we now need to address is how, in the work we ask GPs to do, we ensure maximum use of their expensive scientific training. A radical answer would be to decide that scientific medical training is to be used for dealing with medical problems only, and that everything else that currently finds its way into GP surgeries – social and economic problems, problems requiring personal counselling and so on – are to be 'treated' by social workers, health visitors, psychologists, counsellors and the like. These professionals, along with GPs, could form 'health' teams operating screening systems to diagnose problems and direct patients along an appropriate treatment pathway. Such a system would deliver a better health care service and allow GPs to do the job they've actually been trained for. The leadership of such a team would be an issue though because although many practices even now work as teams, the members of it who are not doctors are still very much at the base of the power pyramid while the doctors are at the top. I can't see doctors giving up that position.

Retirement has taken me from provider to recipient of health care. As I watch the changes continue – illness becoming 'sickness' and patients becoming 'customers' and 'clients' – I sometimes feel that I'm losing my bearings! My view of what patients should be able to expect of their general practitioner remains *unchanged*, however, and can still be summed up by the three 'C's – competence, continuity of care and compassion. Sadly, none of these can be guaranteed these days – for a variety of reasons. Competence, for example, seems as variable as ever, though I would suspect that, with all the quality training now available, attitude rather than ignorance may be the explanation there. As to providing continuity of care, the enormous increase in sessional and part-time GP contracts seriously undermines that aspiration. It also has the effect of making truly compassionate, personal care very difficult to deliver: it's not unusual now for a patient to have to relate to more than one doctor during a course of treatment.

The significant increase in the financial reward made to GPs in recent times and the increase in power which many have achieved through fund-holding have also, in my view, contributed to a weakening of the notion of general practice as a vocation, and this too, affects doctor-patient relationships: I think we may come to regret these changes.

Would I do medicine again? I don't know. I always had a yen to be a teacher at a boarding school where I could be involved in the whole life of the place – the social life, athletics and so on. I think I would have enjoyed that. So I'm not sure that medicine *was* my proper vocation, but I did it, and I've no regrets.

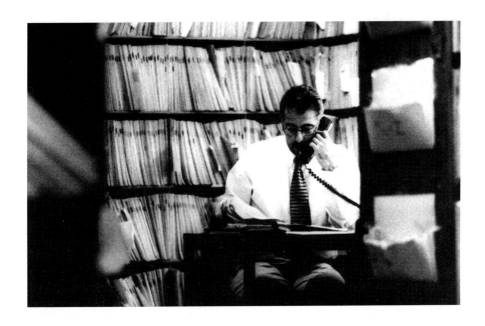

9

My father was a GP. He came from a poor family in Leeds and got a scholarship to go to university. When he qualified just after the war general practice was very different from how it is now: he set up as a single-handed GP in a very deprived part of the city by putting a plaque up at the door and waiting for patients to turn up. As a child I admired him very much. I was also aware of the amount of pleasure that he got out of his work; he was a very, very committed Socialist who had strong beliefs and moral codes which he lived by. I don't feel that I was ever pushed, but I was bright, and becoming a doctor just seemed the right thing to do. And it had to be general practice; I never really thought of anything else.

I came to university in Scotland and have been here ever since. Being a junior doctor was just tiring and exhausting. People at you all the time. It's not a lot about medicine: there's a lot of form filling and blood taking and getting up in the middle of the night to deal with very trivial things and it's very, very hard work. But once I'd got that all out of the way, I really felt that I was now general practice bound and every job I did was interesting: I knew that everything I was learning would be useful one day. I knew too that I wanted to work in a deprived area; my father had instilled into me that if you had something to offer you should do as much as you could with it, so I chose to do my trainee year in another area of the city rather like this and it was a fantastic time – very good training, good people, good job. It was like finding the end of the rainbow I suppose, something that I'd always wanted to do and then one day I was there – I had a desk and I was a GP (well, a trainee GP!) and it just felt right, that this was where I should be. It was a wonderful environment; my colleagues were incredibly supportive and caring, the sort of people that I felt in tune with. They were there because they wanted to be there, saying the things that I wanted to hear. It was very exciting – everything I'd hoped for; and then I failed to get a qualified GP job! So I did a year as a geriatric registrar, which was very enjoyable even though it wasn't what I wanted to do. And then this job came up; I've been here eleven years now. It's an area of multiple deprivation, and I'm one of seven doctors serving 9,500 patients: an average practice would have four doctors for that number. Much of our time is spent dealing with minor, self-limiting illness – coughs, sore throats and so on – but we also see a huge amount of psychiatric problems, drug problems, and drug-associated problems.

There's an immediacy about our patients' health care needs which is always there: everything has to be done *now*, *where* they want it and *when* they want it and often that's not tomorrow and not even this evening, and it has to be a house call rather than in the surgery and so on. I think this is all because their GPs are one of the few groups of people that they have power over. Lots of people, lots of organisations have let deprived people down; it's easy to imagine them saying, 'My parents let me down; I'm in a crappy house, the Housing's let me down; I'm not getting enough money, the DSS has let me down; the Social Worker I used to have has left and I don't like the new one, so Social Work has let me down,' and so on. General Practice tends to be a constant: if you choose, it can be constant for almost the whole of your life. You can ring the Housing up and say, 'I want a new house' and be told, 'Sorry you'll have to wait.' Or you can ring the DSS up and say, 'I need some more money' and be told, 'Sorry, you're not entitled to more.' But if you ring up your GP and say, for example, 'I need an appointment now – I think I've got meningitis,' nobody's going to say, 'I'm sorry, we can't see you'; or if you ring up your GPs and say, 'My daughter's unconscious. Please get here now!' of course we will go. I don't believe our patients operate a malicious angry powerbase: I think rather that they look to us for support and know we will give it. It's about trust. Our patients are amazingly trusting and honest and open: they know that they can always see us and they know that we'll be honest and decent with them, so therefore they use us.

In an area like this, it's very important for a doctor to try to maximise patients' income, because research has shown that the richer you are, the healthier you are. So when I fill in forms which report that patients have certain illnesses which entitle them to benefits they would not otherwise get, I feel I'm genuinely helping. And when patients get these little bits of extra money they may find life more bearable: my hope is that as a result they will also become healthier. Dealing with the links between poverty and ill-health by trying to provide more money is no different, to me, from seeing a patient with pneumonia and prescribing antibiotics: in each situation, I'm simply giving appropriate treatments. Just as certain medicines are appropriate treatments for particular diseases, so more money, or holidays or a better house may also improve my patient's health. This may be seen as a subversive view but I don't make the decisions about which people, in the end, actually *get* extra money or a better house; I just use my professional expertise to provide information for those who make the decisions, and naturally I'm very happy to do that because I think my patients may benefit.

I have a theory however that very poor people can see illness as a very positive thing; not only does it give a certain status, it can open up an entitlement to benefits. I'm not jumping on the DSS scrounger bandwagon here: I just believe that if, for example, somebody who is poor has epilepsy which entitles him to a disability living allowance, then in a way epilepsy is a good thing to have, and the person is quite happy to talk about his fits. I even think that sometimes, for very poor people, ill health may give an increased sense of identity. That probably sounds a pretty dreadful thing to say – almost incredible in fact – but if someone's living in dreadful poverty and they're told that if they have three fits a week they'll get a certain amount of extra money but if they have only one fit a week they won't get any extra money, it's not difficult to see the appeal of having the three fits. Unfortunately there's a corollary to this however: just because ill-health may in this complicated way be seen as beneficial, many people around here may, I fear, suffer ill health more willingly than they should, and this in turn creates for *us* a battle against chronic illness which we will perhaps never really win unless we deal with the issues of poverty, identity, self-belief and so on.

The preventable ill health in this area is enormous, and we know that there are strategies which could prevent it: I don't think however that this practice has the power to change much of people's ill-health, even though the political will is there. I feel an enormous amount of anger that GPs have been told to look after most of the 'health' of the nation, especially when what I'm having to do is very different from what a GP in a more affluent part of the city is doing. Government health targets are unrealistic for this area; images of health that focus on not smoking and drinking less than 21 units of alcohol a week and having a healthy diet and taking exercise refer to a different population. The targets are technically to do with my patients because of course they are, for example, at higher risk, but to just blandly say we want a 30% reduction in these conditions without accepting that there are specific needs in areas like this which must also be tackled, is unrealistic. If you want to overtake 'Health for the Nation' targets in this sort of area you have to adopt a different approach: you can't expect primary care to deliver everything – that's impossible, absolutely impossible. We find it difficult enough looking after our patients' day-to-day medical problems without looking after every risk they have as well. 'Health' strategies require funding and resources.

GPs are, of course, increasingly expected to look after the finances of the Health Service too. I find it very, very difficult to not only prioritise among my patients and their individual problems, but also to prioritise them within the context of what's happening in the rest of the city and the rest of the UK. I agree that my patients' needs must be set within a wider context but I don't think it's up to *me* to worry about the patient who is sitting in the next room or the next practice. If I want my patient to have coronary artery bypass surgery my view is that I need to fight as hard as I can to get it and my patient needs to know that I can be trusted to do that. I don't think that trust will be there if my patient knows that I'm balancing up four other patients with him, I don't know how much money I've got in my kitty and maybe x is more important than y. I think I should be referring and pleading for my patient only, and somebody with an overview should be deciding priorities. Maybe that person will say, 'We're very sorry, but your 53 year old unemployed man with no kids will have to wait eight weeks for a by-pass because we've decided that the 45 year old employed man with two kids who at the moment is not able to go to work because of his heart condition needs priority treatment'. If they do I will have to live with that, but as long as priorities are worked out properly on principles I agree with that's fine. I think the patients will then have faith in me and I can have faith in the system. Fund-holding destroyed any faith I had. There needs to be a public debate on rationing and prioritising.

Having said all that, I think the purchaser/provider split has been very important: the changes which have allowed us to know what we're doing within the NHS, to realise that there is an issue about resources and priorities and that money is not infinite are very important. And it's good that within the NHS now there are certain ways in which my patients' needs *can* be prioritised.

Prioritising and rationing are, of course, not new concepts: we've always let patients suffer and even die in this country. In America private medicine does everything to maximise profits of organisations and to try to maximise the health of the patients too; these two strands, however, do not always run hand-in-hand. We don't do that here. We don't offer everybody everything: we prioritise every single day, and we *must* do that. Ironically, the evidence is that, in general terms, we're as healthy as the Americans are – and probably healthier in many ways because we don't do things for people which are useless or unnecessary but profitable. And we're cheaper too. So I accept rationing, it's just that as a GP working here, I feel that I must continue to work for the interests of my patients all the time. That's partly because I know that the demands of the more articulate, more intelligent people in society are always heard, whereas our patients, because they're very passive, inarticulate, are *not* heard; so I must be their advocate – I think our patients especially deserve that because they have no other advocates. I'm happy to fill the advocate's role, but I can't be the rationer as well. If the resources of the NHS need looking after there are people with much more appropriate knowledge and a much better strategic overview than me who should decide priorities.

I would suspect that a GP from a prosperous area who came and worked here for a week would seriously question whether I was doing my job properly, because it wouldn't be recognisable. In more prosperous areas life is much more straightforward; patients can read and write, they probably consulted for some advice, they can read the prescription, they probably *will* go to the chemist and get it, they probably will take it properly. The scope of general practice is meant to be infinite, but here everything is magnified. We're no doubt doing things here that practices in better-off areas wouldn't be doing, but it seems to me important – absolutely vital in fact – that we operate as we do. We're simply being patient-centred; that, for me, is as it should be. The pressure is on us of course to be harassing people to come in for cholesterol and blood pressure checks; well, we could spend the same amount of time doing that, but we'd have to employ another seven doctors to do it, and the success rate would be small. That's one of the frustrating things about our situation here; we do what we do quite well, but it takes up a lot of our time and prevents us doing other things which we could be doing which we know can improve health.

Communities like this tend to get a very good deal one to one from general practice because on the whole they're looked after by very caring people who make the decision to work in such areas, but they do miss out on other aspects of health care. The truth is that for really poor, deprived people, achieving good health is a very low priority; their lives are so full of very stressful, very immediate, very demanding medical/social problems that as their GP you are left with very little time to deal with cardiovascular risks or ischaemic heart disease risks or cancer risks or sexual health: all these things that middle-class people are able to tune in to just aren't really focused for poor people because every minute of their day is involved in much more basic concerns. I've always felt that if I worked in an affluent area I could put up a notice saying 'Get your child immunised' or 'Have your smear done' or 'Come and have your cholesterol measured', and there would be a queue at the door. Here we have to send out hundreds of appointments and reminders and re-reminders and spend time writing letters and visiting people simply to get a basic level of health screening, like smears, done at all. I would say that in a practice like this we work three times harder to achieve half the results for health promotion, and you've got to have different strategies for reaching people. We do achieve our targets, but only because we employ a lot of staff and everyone makes a huge effort.

I find my work incredibly stressful some of the time. Minute after minute, hour after hour, day after day, it's very, very wearing *giving* all the time; sometimes it's all too much. There are individual things – like patients who are occasionally aggressive – which I think we all find difficult, and then there are the constant demands for help with problems not specifically about health. Apart from the whole range of low level illness and other problems I've mentioned, we also spend a lot of time on our patients' behalf dealing with social workers wanting to consult, with the DSS, the police and the courts. It amazes me how important we must be to some people – go to the doctor, get a letter, problem solved. There are no boundaries here to what a doctor could be asked to help with: I suspect we're the new priests. Today for example we've had five phone calls so far from a patient whose partner is in police custody. She wants him released because he's got a bad back and she's been told by her lawyer that if we give her a letter describing his medical condition the police will let him out. I've had to put it to her that we don't think we should respond like that; we agree he's got a bad back, and we'll mention it if his lawyer or the police want to contact us; but the phone calls have continued all day. I do understand the problem: this woman is obviously very needy: her partner's in the cells and she wants him out. But maintaining sympathy, empathy with that problem despite the fact that you've had five phone calls and you really want to get on with something else, is very difficult.

You have to learn to protect yourself from the very high levels of stress that you're exposed to as a GP. People do this in different ways; some turn into pure clinicians, just dealing unemotionally with the problems, while other people try to take on everything and find it too difficult. In this practice we probably all manage to find a path which is comfortable. I probably instil some dependency in my patients; I do want to please and that tends to take the form of inviting them to get back in touch with me if there's anything I can do (and of course there's always *something* I can do), but that's what's comfortable for me. Even as a trainee I was much more interested in talking, in psycho-social dynamics, consultation techniques, wider ideas about illness and health in the context of people's lives and so on than in learning through dealing with the coughs and colds and sore throats!

The rewards of my job are to do with the role I'm given here, with knowing that I do have an importance in people's lives, and also the power to make a difference. As a doctor here you're truly a part of a community where people know every one of their neighbours and everyone knows you too. You see people meeting up at the shopping arcade, you meet them showing off their newborn children to everyone and so on: I think it's fantastic to be part of that. Earlier today I went into the baker's and did an impromptu consultation because the woman behind the counter asked my advice, and then somebody came in with their new baby and we all admired the baby and talked about that. The feeling of being part of my patients' lives – not just visiting them in their homes but in a wider way too – is very touching. I sometimes think how awesome their trust is; so long as you treated people here with kindness and consideration and respect they would believe you were doing them good – even if you were actually quite weak clinically. We're probably more important in the lives of some of our patients than anyone would ever imagine; they relate to us very much as people did in my father's day – respecting the doctor's judgement and trusting him to make you well if he possibly can. When a new doctor comes it's the talk of the place.

Most people who work in areas like this have made a positive decision to come here, and that makes for a very supportive working environment. You have lots of strings to your bow, so your professional life is very fulfilling. I couldn't see myself in hospital medicine apart perhaps from cancer care or geriatrics or psychiatry – all very patient-centred areas of work. But I still don't think any of that would match this; I couldn't see it matching this at all. I expect to stay here; after 11 years I feel I'm getting quite good at my job. I'll probably reach a peak soon, though, and I don't know what might happen then. I hope that I would have the capacity to reconsider what I was doing if I ever began to get stale; I could never go on doing this job if I lost interest in it – for me it *is* a vocation.

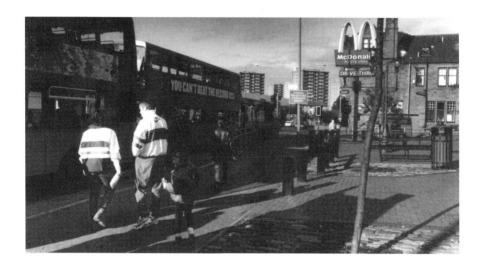

Inner City

10

Female GP
Graduated 1981
Location: Deprived inner city practice

My family came to Scotland from Poland. My mother trained as a doctor, but didn't practise after she moved here. I didn't intend to do medicine; as a teenager I was interested in science and did my first degree in Virology and Immunology. Deciding to be a doctor came later, and my sister helped fund me through medical school. Over the course of my medical studies it became apparent to me that general practice offered the greatest variety of work, contact with people and career flexibility and so, because I knew that I wanted to have a family as well as a job, I decided that this was the way to go. I did my training in a very posh urban practice. We had occasional forays into the bad bits of the city, but it was essentially a wealthy area.

The practice I've been in since then – inner-city, massively impoverished – couldn't be more different from where I trained, though the full extent of the deprivation wasn't completely apparent to me at first. I remember driving around counting the number of alsatians and burnt-out houses because I thought that this would be a pretty good index of what the neighbourhood was like. But the appearance of the place fooled me; there were fewer burnt-out houses than I expected, but what I didn't know was that unlike other places I'd been, where setting fire to your house was a way of getting re-housed somewhere better, housing in this area was zero-rated and nobody wanted it, so if you burned your house down you were simply re-housed in another awful building round the corner. It was all, in reality, far worse than anything I'd ever seen.

There are three of us here for 4,000 patients. A lot of the housing has been cleared recently, and our list size has dropped because of that. One of the things that attracted me to this practice was the very positive attitude of the other partners to the community and to the team philosophy; though I work part-time I've always felt included in all the decision-making. I used to do a lot of family planning work but I've gradually branched out from that to psycho-sexual counselling; I trained with the Institute of Psycho-Sexual Medicine. For some time I was also deputy Trainer for the practice, and became the main trainer in 1997. Becoming a Training Practice was a massive undertaking, but it's been a good development; we're all committed to it and it's improved the standard of service we deliver by constantly making us question what we do.

The practice has quite a high profile in the community. My partner got an MBE some time ago for his work with drug addicts; I think we're known as a practice that's fairly tolerant of difficult patients. A lot of our work is typical of a poor area – minor childhood illnesses and diseases related to poverty and stress. Incidences of heart disease, lung cancer, chronic respiratory disease and duodenal ulcer are well above the national average. There are also many more patients with diabetes and rheumatoid arthritis. There's a higher than average incidence of premature death from heart disease, with young families left and so on; in general, the mortality rates here for patients under 65 are twice that of prosperous areas. On the other hand we do have people who are physically tough and live to 80 or even 90. I think there's a kind of natural selection going on; those that survive the usual killers keep going for ever!

Drug and alcohol addiction are huge problems in this area. A majority of our patients will have had one or more of the addiction problems somewhere along the line, but we don't ban addicts from the practice so long as they admit to their problem. In general the addicts we treat are manageable and don't threaten us; they occasionally cause a rumpus, but that's comparatively rare. We do try to treat them with respect, but we expect respect in turn, so that if they want to be seen they have to turn up as agreed, to an ordinary appointment, on time. If they do that we'll discuss things properly with them. Unfortunately, the down-side of our policy on addiction is that we've become known as a practice with a lot of addicts, and that sometimes scares more 'normal' patients away.

Our prescribing statistics are completely distorted by regular prescriptions for methadone. They're also distorted by large numbers of people on benefits coming to the practice for free prescriptions for even very simple things like paracetamol and Calpol. When there's a flu epidemic here we'll have up to 70 people at a surgery wanting paracetamol! Prescriptions of this kind are a pretty good indicator of the poverty of an area; prosperous people wouldn't dream of wasting their time coming for them; they'd just go and buy the medication themselves.

The social problems here are huge. I got funding some years ago for a project looking at the demand for counselling, and we actually thought we'd uncover a lot of problems to do with direct effects of poverty – housing, financial issues, divorce and so on. Well, these certainly did come up, but to a lesser extent than I'd expected; people often know they're in a poverty trap and don't need to discuss it. But the problems that did come up really threw us; a large number of our patients had a history of abuse, and there was also a lot of unresolved grief. This was often linked to the death of a youngish person in circumstances that are not very acceptable socially; if your son dies driving a stolen car, or sniffing glue, or taking a drug overdose, or having contracted AIDS, it's quite difficult to grieve openly and have the support of the community. Deaths that are felt as shameful in some way can become a terrible psychological burden to a family. Death through suicide has a similar effect.

It's not all grim here, though; there are also families in which there's a strong spirit of support – probably fewer than in the past, though, as a lot of the most motivated skilled working class families that were in this area have moved out. Years ago a lot of men round here worked on the railway and in the locomotive works, but in the 1960s a lot of other very run-down areas of the city were cleared and families dumped here. But with the older people you still go into houses where the grandchildren's graduation photographs are prominently displayed and they're lawyers and doctors and so on. That can bring its own pressures for the practice of course because sometimes these younger members of the family who've advanced educationally and socially come to visit granny and start stirring things because they think she should be in a better environment, even though granny would be like a fish out of water in a posh part of town. Having said that, there are also really sad and difficult situations where a respectable elderly couple may be left in a close that has filled up with very undesirable families and it's like getting through a war-zone trying to reach them. That is awful.

The unemployment rate here is horrendous; it affects everything including, even, the children's schooling. If there's no one regularly in work in a household, it's difficult to pressure children to attend school regularly, or to organise yourself to get up in the morning and see that they do. There's a lot of moonlighting goes on but I would estimate that less than 30% of people here are in any form of proper work. I resist labelling but I'd have to admit that much of the population here does fit the profile of an underclass – people who don't have a work ethic, who don't get married because it's economically unviable, whose relationships break down because of the problems of deprivation. We also have patients who have maybe three children with different surnames and none of the fathers permanently resident in the house because of the effect that would have on benefits. You also find matriarchal families of four or five generations – great-granny, granny, mother and daughters and so on – where the men seem to have completely vanished from the house. They may re-appear occasionally, but they don't really form part of the family unit. Some of the men here are still in adolescent gangs at the age of 30.

The problems among children and young teenagers are very worrying. We see seven and eight year olds with behaviour problems, grotty diets and grotty teeth and feel powerless to stop it all happening. And then there's the under-age pregnancies – despite real efforts on the part of the practice to educate, provide contraception and so on. I don't condone under-age sex, but since I'm conscious that it's happening anyway I try to make it as easy as possible for young people to get contraceptives. I have various ploys – for example if I have a 13 or 14 year old girl coming in for antibiotics I'll mention that certain kinds sometimes don't work so well if the person is on the contraceptive pill. If they say they're not I take the opportunity to mention that if they ever need it they should just let me know. A lot of the girls are very sensible but some clearly are involved in very early sexual relationships from which pregnancies do often result. I was shocked when I first came here that I was never asked to arrange abortions. I'm a Catholic but I've never let that interfere with how I advise patients. In my prosperous training practice requests for abortion were quite common, but here the girls often just keep the baby. They don't seem to be able to make any kind of conscious decision about their pregnancy and often try to ignore it until it is very obvious to all around.

We've always believed in health promotion in this practice though we haven't always approved of the way it's been specified. We try to focus on health issues with patients – about things like child-rearing, improving diet and so on – but a lot of our patients are quite anti 'groups' and find them very threatening. We've been trying to set up a food co-operative and look at eating habits, but people here are not very daring and it's difficult to get them to try new things. I think it requires quite a lot of self-esteem to branch out in all sorts of ways and a lot of our patients don't have that confidence. We were involved some time ago in a scheme to raise awareness of heart disease where you fed in a lot of information about patients' lifestyle and so on, but we had to tread very carefully as some of our patients ended up with predictions of almost 100% likelihood of dying within the next five years. They were so shocked they just went out and lit up another cigarette. It really didn't help, and it certainly traumatised the investigators who'd been putting the information in. That example just demonstrates one problem we have with health promotion schemes, which is that it would never occur to the people setting them up how people in an area like this might be affected by them. The whole health promotion issue needs to be programmed differently for different populations.

The same is true of health promotion publications. Years ago there were some very good, very straightforward leaflets which just showed you what nourishment you got from common foods – fish fingers, porridge, fruit and so on. These have now been replaced by very gimmicky leaflets which have, for example, kiwi fruits on legs hopping off the page. That doesn't mean anything to our patients because most of them don't know what a kiwi fruit is. And there's no way that I'm suddenly going to get people here to start eating red bean casseroles either – for the same reason. These materials just don't engage our patients; if all you have to offer is fancy pictures of things they've never considered eating anyway, you're not going to change their habits. The gulf is huge. Big, stylish health education campaigns completely miss the point in areas like this; small, sharply focused practical initiatives are much more effective. I'd like to see more very basic cookery classes going on. That would mean that I could say to my patient, 'Why not go round the corner to so and so, they're there every week. Go and pay your £1 and you'll be shown how to make a good meal out of it.' That's the educational level we need to be operating on.

There are lots of social and psychological pressures on poor families too, which create a lot of stress. This is the kind of area where your kid gets hassle if they don't have the right kind of £80 trainers, or the right jacket or jeans. This results in people way down in the social pecking order trying to find the money for these kinds of status symbols, but you can bet, with unemployment as high as it is here, that most of that isn't going to be found legally.

It's also a constant struggle for parents to keep their children safe here, because the peer pressure is all towards anti-social behaviour, violence, law-breaking. I saw a wee boy of nine recently who'd been virtually rejected by his mother and her new partner because he just wasn't like other kids. He didn't like playing out in the street trying to set fire to cars and schools. He preferred to sit and read. His grandmother who brought him along was terribly worried about him. She wanted me to send him to a psychiatrist to get him sorted out because he wasn't out there kicking the shit out of the slightly smaller boy in the street. And when he got hit by the other boys he came in and didn't fight back or sneak out a knife and scar somebody. It's a shocking case, and yet the granny's attitude was understandable; she believed he wasn't going to survive secondary school unless he changed. And you could see that she had a point; within the community the boy wasn't 'normal'. But you can imagine how I felt writing a referral letter: '...This child doesn't fit in. He doesn't set fire to cars, isn't violent in expected ways. Please can you help...?'

I find it terribly sad the way areas like this have gone over the years; when you talk to older people you hear about the pigeons they've kept or the dogs they've run or the various sports they've been involved in. So many young people round here now have virtually no aspirations, and at the same time they regard so many of the things that older people did as having a definite 'working class' label attached, so they wouldn't be seen dead doing them. The irony is that these older people got genuine feelings of success and self-respect from their hobbies, felt proud of their achievements. There is very little that many of the young people round here now can find any satisfaction in, or indeed could be trusted to do; you can't, for example, put them in to help old ladies, because they would probably steal their pension book. I believe that some of the girls resort to having a child because they imagine they'll somehow be good at that – but of course if they haven't been good at anything else so far, and particularly if they've had pretty poor parenting themselves, it's unlikely that they will make a success of it.

There are many, many young people suffering from stress and depression in this area. Many break down or attempt suicide. One national project measuring levels of illness and distress in various parts of Scotland indicates that this area has an attempted suicide incidence substantially higher than the average. Another problem we have here is trying to support young mothers who have a history of abuse or drug addiction in their own background and who therefore need a great deal of support in dealing with their own children, to try to prevent illness or abuse occurring.

We get quite a number of travelling families on our patch. I feel that they often get quite a rough deal from the health services. Some doctors won't take them on as permanent patients and treat them instead as temporary residents which means they do get emergency treatment, but they never get any continuity in terms of care or health promotion and they hardly ever get any proper medical records. Sometimes they're seen at a hospital and there's no record of it. We've made it our policy to take travellers on as patients so that they can actually benefit from call-ups for checks and so on, but they often can't read or write so we have to go chasing them up.

You have to be very flexible if you want to persuade people round here – travellers or residents – to come into the health system. In terms of looking after the health of children we make a big effort on immunisations, but we often only succeed because our Health Visitors have chased patients to get them. And with the adults: one of my colleagues decided to set up a Well Woman Clinic and sent out fifty invitations; two people replied, one made an appointment and in the end nobody showed up. So many people are just too disorganised to get themselves here. We need to keep reminding ourselves how different our patients' lives are; hardly anyone in the area would be likely to have a diary; they will sometimes stick pins into the wall with reminders, but if they then move house between appointments that's pretty hopeless. So there's a lot of extra work by clerical and nursing staff just to get people organised to have any health care at all.

Mammography rates are pretty low here, and there's a contingent of women in their 50s who resist having cervical smears in case it shows up cancer. There's quite a widespread head-in-the-sand attitude; people just don't want to know if they've got something serious. Women are better at coming along if, say, they find a breast lump, but the other side of their deciding that this is the moment to come to the surgery is that they can then be quite demanding, wanting a doctor now and not in a day or two. We try to guarantee an appointment within three working days but often that's not good enough for them and patients can be quite abusive. When it's appropriate I will sometimes point out that they've admitted they've had their problem for three months but today's the first we've heard about it. In those circumstances it doesn't seem unreasonable that they should wait a day or two until I can deal with it properly.

Because of the terrible social situation here, we find ourselves under pressure to deal with a lot of problems which, if you really examine them, are not really medical at all. We get children brought in with sickness and diarrhoea and a demand that we should see them right away and perhaps in the background what's driving the mother is that the washing machine is broken and she can't wash clothes and this is all too much; she may even know deep down that she can account for the child being unwell because of something he's been allowed to eat. Another scenario is that if you're a mother with a boyfriend who's likely to hit you when he's annoyed and your child is crying constantly and won't go to sleep and you can see the boyfriend's level of irritation is rising, again you may well summon the GP to do something even if there's really nothing much wrong with the child.

We spend a lot of time here unravelling the background to situations and trying to judge what's really going on. I have worked with doctors who have told people with social problems to go and see someone else, and refused to be drawn in – and if you try hard enough you can actually switch off during a consultation – but in this practice we try to find out what's behind things that come up. For example, you can't have a mother bring a child with a simple cold to you five times in a few days and not ask yourself why this is happening. I've been accused of being a frustrated social worker, but quite frankly I don't enjoy doing social work; I want to do medicine. I like getting my hands dirty and doing exciting things. I don't think, however, that you can afford to lose sight of the impact of these awful social situations on people's health; whether or not *I* should be the one dealing with these background problems is another issue though. The only alternative we have is to ensure that the practice is providing very easy access to social workers, counsellors or other support workers; it's no use here if that kind of help is even a bus ride away.

We try to encourage people who work in the support services to come and talk to us so that we know what's available for our patients. We see building up links as a good investment because then we can say to people, 'Why not go along the corridor and talk to R—. I know her and I think you'd find that helpful'. Research done by the Scottish Office has shown that when people from the support agencies are located within a practice the patients perceive them as offering the same 'confidential' service as doctors and are more willing to talk to them. Otherwise many people are very shy of going to the statutory agencies. As the doctor you have to be very careful about the confidentiality issue in relation to other professionals, but it does seem to be a helpful arrangement for discussing problems.

As well as providing advice services, we also run groups here for single mums and people with mental health problems. We used to have a social worker in the team but she's been withdrawn because of cuts. Similarly we used to have a counsellor here, financed through short-term funding. Again, that funding has now been withdrawn; a practice with 4000 patients isn't regarded as big enough to support a counsellor. We've continued to support her ourselves though, and we're hoping to be able to manoeuvre money to help cover the cost, because we feel that in the longer term it's a good investment. Unfortunately the benefits don't show up right away – your drug bills don't suddenly drop.

We've had representatives from the Citizens Advice Bureau here talking to people about Welfare Benefit problems and a counsellor from the city's Council on Alcohol also comes here one afternoon as week – so we are trying to develop comprehensive services. A lot of the initiative, however, comes in the end from us making suggestions to the team and people being willing to accommodate what's going on – lending their consulting room for example when they're not there. It's all individual initiatives and I can't help thinking that if it could be properly co-ordinated we could achieve much more.

People still look at me slightly horrified when I say where I work, and the police, when they find out what I do, say things like, 'You don't go out on your own surely?' Well, of course I do, and, in fact, nothing very dramatic has ever happened to me. Having said that I have had a few tense moments however. Someone once offered me some 'free plastic surgery', but she wasn't serious; it was really all just verbal abuse. There have also been occasional situations which have seemed quite menacing but which have ended quite amusingly. For example, in my early days here I was once using a very small consulting room late in the day when most of the reception staff had left, and a big, heavily built drug addict came in and asked for drugs for somewhat unrealistic withdrawal symptoms that I knew he wasn't having, as he'd just got out of prison a few days before. I pointed this out to him and told him there was no way I was going to write him a prescription. He stood up (and I knew he'd been in prison for grievous bodily harm) and said, 'Well, I get violent if I don't get anything,' and I thought that this was the moment of truth. I was so annoyed with him however – I suppose because I felt that he was trying to blackmail me – that I told him to 'piss off' and he just smiled very nicely at me and said, 'Well, you were the new doctor so it was worth a try!' That was it; he smiled and walked out. I was left shaking slightly, wondering how I'd got away with it. He's still around and still smiles nicely to me and has never tried to con me again, but I know I was lucky that it *was* a try on!

For a while there was a perception of inner-city practice as a kind of dead-end job that people who couldn't get something better would settle for and that attitude irritated me very much. No one who works here is in general practice for the money, but equally we're not here because there's nowhere else to go. All of us are very well qualified and could easily get other jobs, but we choose to stay here; we want to provide as good a service to this community as they would get in the leafy suburbs.

There are problems of course; it's harder for a practice to be very efficient in an area where people don't keep appointments, don't have telephones, forget re-call appointments and move addresses every couple of months depending on which money lender's leaning on them. With a lot of work you can achieve your targets though. Yes, it's a lot of hassle, but I find it very rewarding to be able to prove that a practice can be effective in a very deprived area. Our patients are generally very appreciative and don't just take us for granted.

A big irony is that any progress we make here shows as lower incidences of existing problems and so, in terms of applying for resources, we are victims of our own success. We're trying to improve things by working on record-keeping which allows us to describe a number of problems which a patient may have. By doing this we are now at least getting some harder data which will help us argue our case for resources, though that's not without its problems too, because when you're fighting for your share of resources in an area, it's your own colleagues in nearby practices that you're competing with.

The staffing issue in general practice isn't just about clinical staff – it's about everyone from receptionists to doctors. Our staff are very loyal to the practice and have coped with a lot of change, but everyone is under a lot of stress. Receptionists in particular are in the front line, dealing with distressed or disturbed or threatening patients, patients who are drunk or high on drugs and so on. They get a lot of abuse. I'm not sure I would cope as well if I were a receptionist here; unlike doctors, receptionists can't be rude back.

The whole tenor of general practice has changed enormously in the last thirty years; GPs used to be generalists dealing with a multitude of clearly defined illnesses – pneumonia, TB, acute infections and so on. Nowadays patients are very unlikely to die of acute illness in their 40s and 50s and our official profile is very much more that of family physicians dealing with preventive medicine, screening, and long term care of the chronically ill. Unfortunately, however, general practice is still one of the few community services that's available 24 hours a day free of charge and since it's very acceptable socially to go to the doctor we do tend more and more to get all kinds of problems dumped on us – social problems, financial problems, problems that in the past the priest or the minister would have dealt with. I really don't know if there's any way out of that.

I think one of the reasons I've stayed here so long is that the team – district nurses, health visitors, practice nurses and receptionists as well as GPs – is so committed. It is very easy to get burnt out in an area like this; there are times when I think I'm just hitting my head off a brick wall, but the support within the team is very strong. We now have a meeting once a week where everyone and anyone who's involved in working here gets together to talk about cases and more general issues and give each other feedback and support. It's such an antidote to your own frustration when someone in the team is feeling very upbeat about some aspect of the work; that really helps when you're feeling like jacking it in for good. If it wasn't for the team this would be a disastrously depressing area to work in.

Putting more money into the Health Service itself will not cure the problems we find here; putting more money into employment would be, for me, the right way to go. I dare say that sounds like shooting myself in the foot because there are clearly many needs within the NHS, but I feel that the real needs occur earlier on in a person's life; poor health so often arises from poor diet and lack of self esteem, frequently linked to lack of work. So many people here lead lives of great poverty, stress and difficulty. So many of the men can no longer fulfil the role of provider for their family in any way. These problems have huge, damaging effects on people's lives. So I think if I was invited to direct a sudden massive injection of money into society with the purpose of improving the health of communities like this I'd be putting it into training and work, rather than directly into the NHS.

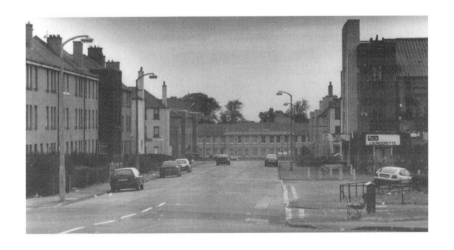

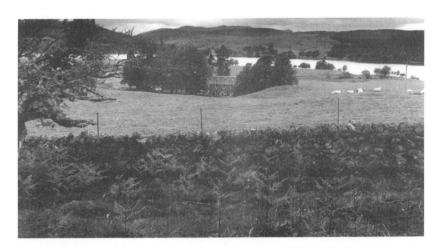

Neighbourhoods

11

Male GP
Graduated 1969
Location: Single-handed remote Highland practice

When I left school I worked first of all as a lab technician in a hospital, but my boss there encouraged me to go and study medicine. I applied to Glasgow University and was duly accepted, and became one of the older students in my year. After about two years in medical school I felt pretty disillusioned however, because I still hadn't come across a patient, and I took a year out. I worked as an uncertificated teacher, but I found teaching too repetitive and eventually went back to university. When I got to the clinical stage of my training things got better because I began to experience what I'd imagined medicine was all about, and I also came to see why we had done so much physics and chemistry and so on first. But it would have helped if people had been more honest with us about what training to be a doctor was really going to be like: I think quite a few people got lost in the initial stages because they hadn't been properly informed about what to expect.

When I graduated I thought at first I'd be a surgeon, but I ended up doing a year of obstetrics instead. That was an appalling rat race, and because I had married as a student, and by then had two children – which created other pressures in my life – I made the decision to move out of hospital medicine. I would have liked, really, to stay and combine obstetrics and paediatrics, but no such job existed: you had to do gynaecology with obstetrics, and that did absolutely nothing for me. I already realised, too, that it was the involvement with people and their families that I really enjoyed, so I decided to become a GP and accepted the offer of a job in the town in central Scotland that my wife came from.

Twenty odd years ago, when I started in general practice, there was no training scheme: one day I was an obstetrician, and the next day I got in the car, drove to the practice for nine o'clock, was given a list of people to see and a room to see them in, and that was it. It's called learning the hard way. My senior partner saw me more or less as an apprentice, though, and he kept me in order. He was pretty straight: every so often he'd take me aside and tell me, 'You've not done that right!' or 'You've upset Mrs. So-and-so!' I learned pretty quickly.

There were three doctors and a part-time nurse in the practice, with about 5,500 patients, two surgeries seven miles apart, no appointment system, and a high demand for home visits. From the patients' point of view it was an excellent arrangement, because they could always be seen, one way or another, on the day they chose, but in the end we *had* to move towards an appointment system to avoid doing surgeries till 8 o'clock at night.

I stayed in that practice for eight years, but when my senior partner died I felt I'd lost my mentor, and was without someone I trusted to bounce ideas off. I also felt awkward with the younger partners who seemed to view general practice more as a business than a vocation. I had various plans in my head for improving things for the patients – better premises and so on – but we couldn't find anywhere suitable and I began to get rather frustrated. Looking back, I think, too, that I became a senior partner too quickly – I hadn't learned to manage people well, and as the practice team got bigger the job became a chore, which is hopeless – medicine should never be just a job, it should be *the* vocation. So although my family were settled, I decided to move, hoping that I might find a new challenge. That was when we came here.

My practice – 800 patients in 440 square miles bounded largely by the snowlines – is one of the smallest and most remote in the central Highlands. We dispense our own drugs, and it's also an 'inducement' practice, which means I'm virtually salaried. Because GPs are paid by the number of patients they serve, I couldn't, on the ordinary pay scale, afford to live and work here at all unless I was already very well off.

The team consists of myself, my wife (a trained nurse) who holds the fort when I'm out on calls, an Associate GP who covers my time off, and two triple-duty nurses. The nurses are pure gold: they take such a range of skills – midwifery, health visiting and district nursing – into my patients' homes. They're a dying breed though; people training now will have nothing like the same level and range of skill; consequently, in the future, patients here won't have the lovely arrangement where everything to do with their health and illness is looked after by the same person from way before they're born. Also, more and more nursing services are being supplied from further away, so that midwives will soon be hospital-based and will have to come out to our community to deal with our patients. Health visiting, too, will most likely be provided from afar, so while nursing services will still be available, they won't have the personal feel you get now with the jobs being done by people in the community that you already know.

The parish minister and the local home helps are also, in my view, important members of the care team. The home helps are magnificent: they're all shepherds' wives, and genuinely caring people, and they make a major contribution to the well-being of my patients. The minister does virtually all the hospital visiting for us: he phones up once a fortnight when he's going to Perth, asks who's in hospital and where he can find them, and goes down to see them. We have no social workers here: they disappeared over the horizon many years ago and haven't been missed. One of the nurses and I do all the counselling, social care and family planning – that's another part of our teamwork. It's old-fashioned medicine here, straightforward and purposeful. We're self-contained and oblivious of the committee work that many of my colleagues seem to find themselves drawn into.

The remoteness and the wide scatter of patients' homes can create problems – in winter I make some very roundabout trips because of roads being blocked with snow – but people are very faithful and patient, because they realise that I put in a lot of effort to look after everyone. On one occasion when I was involved with a home delivery some distance away, things did not go as expected, and I ended up, with my patient, in the maternity hospital in Perth. From the time I was called out to her house to the time I returned was around eight hours. It was also the middle of a flu epidemic and the surgery was very busy, but knowing I was delayed people just accepted that they'd have to wait. Because of the need to maintain confidentiality, unexpected absences by a doctor are never explained, but in a small community like this people tend to be able to work out what's happening at a given time, and I think this increases their tolerance of any inconvenience to themselves. The acceptance that the doctor can't be everywhere at once is probably unique to practices like this.

The work pattern, too, is different from a town practice: because I'm a single-handed GP I'm on duty for much longer spells of time, though obviously I'm not working every minute of that. When I'm on call, too, I'll often have things like gardening or reading or painting the house on the go, and if someone arrives at the door with a problem I just explain that they'll have to accept me as I am, and after a quick scrub I attend to them. People often ask me if it's stressful being single-handed, but it isn't at all. Everyone knows when you're on, and you just build your social life around it. I was once on call for eighteen weeks without any time off and I know that's not good or healthy, but it was necessary and I didn't feel too bad about it.

Stress is not a disease that we recognise in big way here. Maybe it's because I don't recognise it in myself that I don't recognise it in others. When I was in a city practice however, being on call was stressful; doctors who are on call for a large number of patients don't sleep at night, don't eat their meals, are fearful of when the phone will ring again. It's different here because expectations are different. Of course there's the occasional person who *is* demanding, who hasn't yet learned that if I'm twenty miles up the glen it might be another hour or two before I can deal with their problem, but in general people are aware of the nature of my job. And, as I mentioned already, because they may have come a fair distance to the surgery, patients will often wait for me to come back. It's surprising, too, the use that's made of the waiting room at times: last Saturday morning we had a deer management meeting here because, as it happened, an estate owner, a forester, a game-keeper and a ranger had all come to see me. As each person finished their consultation they just went back to the waiting room to continue the discussion. It made a lot of sense as they all live several miles away from each other!

I think we work a lot on mutual consideration here: my patients know they can rely on me to do whatever needs to be done whenever it comes up, but the other side of that is that people really respect my official time off. My half day is a Wednesday, and people do try to avoid breaking into that. They're quite happy to keep their problem, if it's at all possible, till Thursday morning. They're also very aware of my daily pattern of calls, and if they want a house visit, they'll suggest I look in on them when I'm passing that way anyway. Mind you, their stoicism is not always such a good idea: I had a patient some time ago who lived several miles away, and he phoned me one Monday evening saying he'd like me to drop by on the Tuesday when he knew I'd be coming in that direction. When I discovered the problem was quite severe chest pains however, I suggested to him that I should really come and see him right away, and it was just as well I did, because he'd had a heart attack!

In general people here do have a strong spirit of endurance though. Not long after I came a forestry worker with a broken leg called in to see me; he had a full-length plaster cast on, and was walking on crutches. As we came to the end of our chat I offered him a sick note, but he refused this saying that he had just come in to tell me how he was getting on. He worked in the middle of the wood, and he revealed that he was still going to work, with his plaster cast wrapped in a black poly bag. He also had a night job as a barman in the pub which he was continuing to do. Clearly, there was no way he was going to take time off work. It made me recall how, in my previous practice, issuing medical certificates for two weeks at a time for minor back strains was not uncommon, and yet here was a chap refusing to take time off at all, even with a broken leg. A lot of my patients are like that – dogged and determined: they were brought up to work and they enjoy working and won't accept what they see as handouts. This can be a problem sometimes, however, when they won't claim the benefits that they're entitled to.

It's generally a healthy community here. There's no predominant disease – probably because people have come originally from different parts of the country. You get people who've come from mining areas bringing mining diseases, and people from sophisticated areas bringing sophisticated diseases! We get more unusual things too – occasional cases of malaria, for instance, because of the number of people in the area who travel to fairly exotic places.

The children are pretty healthy too. I haven't referred a child to a paediatrician for several years now, and we don't have anyone at the moment with a chronic disease that's going to shorten their life. Several years ago we did have an outbreak of tuberculosis, so we got the mass radiography unit up and x-rayed everybody, but we never found the source. We managed to treat the four young folk affected at home – which temporarily sent our drugs bill away up! That's a side issue though, because they all got better.

The young people here have the usual emotional ups and downs – the teenage discovery of the opposite sex is just the same as anywhere else! Things can be more difficult for young people at that stage in their lives if they don't have the anonymity that a town offers, so over the years I've built up an understanding with our young folk and look after their needs – sex education, contraception and so on. The girls in particular really enjoy embarrassing me during our wee chats by asking all the awkward questions!

I like to think I'm sympathetic and supportive to them all though. We do get the situation where a teenage girl is brought by her father to the surgery and he sits outside while she comes in to talk about family planning. I always ask if the parents know why they're there and, as you can imagine, the answer often is that officially they've got a sore throat! Things are changing though, and most girls nowadays will talk to their mothers about these things – indeed sometimes the mother and daughter will come along together to get their family planning sorted out. Boys aren't quite so open with their mums and dads though!

The family atmosphere here, the fact that most people's lives cross in some way, often helps me in my work. We now have a practice manager who's also part-time school secretary, and this was a great bonus recently when we were asked if we would do rubella vaccinations for the children. We agreed and were allocated funds to cover three sessions – which seemingly is what it usually takes for that number of cases. In fact we did it all in half-a-session and ended up having coffee with the teachers! The nurse and I just went round to the school at the arranged time and the secretary (our manager), who's with the children at playtime, lunchtime and so on, had them all lined up ready and we got straight into it. It went like clockwork simply because all the children knew us and we knew them, so we could guess who was going to be apprehensive and were ready to make a game of it with them. When we phoned up the Health Board and said we'd finished they asked us how we'd managed it so quickly!

Generally, we have a good relationship with the specialist services. I suppose we do tend to work our cases up first, and don't bother them with any kind of rubbish, so that when we think there's a problem and do refer, we get a pretty swift reaction. Sadly, from time to time, you get the tragic diagnosis – the young person who has developed a disease which means they won't be able to go on working, for example – and there can also be care problems associated with chronic illness. If you're in a big centre, the centre can provide some of the answers to the problem of care, but we don't have those resources here, so we have to support ourselves.

On the other hand, I think that's part of the challenge of working here too. One great thing is that you know so many families, so you know how to tap into support for someone when it's needed. Word gets around quickly – it's the Glasgow tenement neighbourliness thing really – and people organise a support system among themselves to accommodate need. I've even known people to give up their home help temporarily if there's some sort of emergency, so that someone else can benefit. You wouldn't get that in a town because no one would know the other demands that were being made on the system.

Although there's not a particularly large elderly population here, we've had a bad year, and have lost quite a few of our older patients: death is not welcome here, but it's coped with. People here respect death greatly, and they respect you, as the doctor, in the midst of it. If somebody dies today, the surgery will be quieter tomorrow, not because people are frightened, but because they try to avoid intruding on you if they can. Having said that, I think it's also true that people here don't dwell on death – they see bereavement as another day of life, and soon pick up the threads again.

One of the roles that you still have as a single-handed rural GP (which you wouldn't encounter these days in a town practice) is that when a patient dies at home, it's usually you, along with the nurse, that lays out the body; sometimes a member of the family will wish to do it – will see it as a last act for a loved one – or they'll do it with you, but usually it's your job. You then sit in on the planning of the funeral. You also attend the funeral and the cup of tea afterwards, and if you don't go, you have to have a good reason, because it's expected: you're regarded as part of the family. If I can't go to a funeral, I always make sure my wife goes in my place.

There's quite a lot of documentation produced by different bodies on how to deal with bereavement, and once when I was on a course I was asked if I would like to be a candidate in a mock oral examination for membership of the Royal College of GPs. I sat in the hot seat and was asked how I would manage the bereavement situation of a woman dying from breast cancer with secondary spread – how I would cope with her husband and two teenage children. My response was that when she died in the place of her choosing I would do a bereavement visit to the family, ensure that other family members were going to be around in the next few weeks and months, and leave them to it. I was informed that this was totally the wrong approach. When I asked why it was wrong, the examiners asked me about counselling and continuing care. My response was that there was the chance with this lady's impending death to plan things – it was not as if she had died unexpectedly. I felt that the family should be helped prepare for her death rather than being seen after it. According to the Royal College, however, I should have involved health visitors, social workers, bereavement counsellors and a number of other health care professionals whose names I can't even remember.

There was a large measure of support for me from my GP colleagues on the course but they were told that if they adopted my approach they would fail the exam. This is where there's a sort of divide in our profession between those of us who practice what we perceive as reasonable care based on common sense and experience, and those who tell us what we should be doing. It's not quite as bad as it used to be, but there are still examination situations where, if you don't follow the Royal College theories, you fail. In my view, the College's theory of bereavement management is inappropriate to my situation because it doesn't take account of life as it really is in a community like this, where the wider community itself, as well as the GP, lends support to individuals in times of need. For example, there's a patient in the practice whose husband died last weekend, and when I was coming down the lochside this morning I passed her coming back from church. Now I know she has coped with the immediate situation, and that her friends are rallying round. She was at church this morning to keep in touch with her community. People here are pretty down to earth and they learn from each other how to manage it all. That doesn't mean to say I'm going to ignore their needs: I'm here if they need me, and I think they know that.

I'm sometimes asked how *I* cope with the deaths of my patients. I'd have to admit that sometimes I just wail! You can't help becoming emotionally involved in a small community like this because often you've known the people so well – they're your friends too. Some situations are particularly difficult; suppose a young man has had a heart attack; you know the ambulance is half an hour away, and you're working hard all that time by yourself, probably down on the floor, to try to keep him going. If he survives, that's a really good feeling; on the other hand, if he dies, you're left sitting there alone with the body – and you sit there and you ask yourself if you really did everything you could for him. That can really get to you.

I've talked about the good relationship we have here, and about how understanding people are. I would say, too, that I feel people respect my judgement, and I don't see the kind of aggression that gets talked about a lot these days. What I do think has changed over the years though is that there's much more of a demand from patients now to know the truth about their condition, so I no longer conceal a diagnosis. If someone has a terminal illness, I'll tell them, and I'll explain what the likely pattern of things will be. You can only really quote statistics of course, but I'll talk it through, and also try to give people options for how their illness might be managed. I decided to do this partly because the hospitals started doing it and then I, as the GP, didn't have a choice; but I think it's right, anyway. What right have I to lie to you? I can think of situations where, if I had lied to my patient, our relationship would have gone down the drain immediately. Many people who are dying want to make plans (plan their funeral even), want to be in control. Often, they seem to set themselves targets – something they've got to stay alive for, like a family wedding or some other important event; I can think of several cases like that we've had here. Once the event is past, the patient often dies quite quickly.

Looking back, I feel that city practice is a grey man existence; you go in at nine in the morning and come home at six, probably to a different part of town, and there's no real contact between you and your patients apart from consultations; deputising services for night calls can only take that separation further. General practice doesn't work that way here; we're part of each others' lives: I hadn't realised, for example, how much my patients cared for *my* welfare until my wife and I went to the Caribbean for a Silver Wedding celebration and got caught up in a hurricane. When we came back my locum said that he'd had more enquiries about our safety than he'd had about people's own health! That wouldn't have happened in a city practice, because people in general wouldn't know anything about their GP's life beyond the surgery.

And it's enriching living here: I'm not the only expert around. I've learned a lot in fifteen years – I know a bit about deer management, forestry, hill farming – just as a lot of my patients know a bit about my work. Knowing each other as people helps us empathise with each other's situations. One of the things that seems to me to be missing now is the opportunity for medical students to experience the reality of other kinds of jobs; because I needed the money when I was a student, I worked every holiday – on building sites, in shipyards, in hospitals and so on. (I was a ward orderly one summer, so I can also count making beds and putting on a decent bandage among my skills!) The main outcome though was that I learned a lot about how other people live and think, and I learned to respect other ways of life. Looking back, I believe it was a really valuable experience for me for my future life as a doctor, particularly for working in a rural practice like this where good trusting relationships and the ability to live in a group are really important.

There's been a lot of change in the time I've been here. Although the population in size is the same, quite a number of people have come and gone. Sometimes people come here because they imagine it will be their ideal environment, but they find it's not so easy and only stay for a year or two. Others do stay and become very much part of the community, accepting the local culture and its idiosyncrasies. And then of course there are the people who *were* born here or have lived here a very long time – hill farmers, foresters and so on – and they're living a life not that different from what you'd have found at the turn of the century.

Some years ago there was a chap at the far end of the loch – a shepherd – I used to shoot with. He had angina and I was trying to get him to slow down a bit but he didn't have time for that. His son and grandson were up staying with him and his wife, and they decided to go fishing up on one of the hill lochs. He took them part of the way up the hill on the tractor and arranged to wait for them. Some hours later they came back from the fishing and the tractor was there but there was no sign of him. When they went to the sheep pen on the hill they found him sitting upright against the dyke with the dog in his lap, and he was dead. He'd finished clipping the sheep, had sat down to eat his sandwiches, and had just died.

They brought him down the hill in a box on the back of the tractor and I was called to the house. In the strict sense of the law, he shouldn't have been moved from his place of death, but what could we do about it? His wife knew that he'd been living on the edge, and she felt he couldn't have died in a nicer way – that he'd have been pleased with his death. She wanted to lay him to rest herself – they'd talked about it and that was their wish – so I ended up keeping Granny company in the kitchen. I made tea for us all – which tickled Granny – and we sat around together and spoke about A–'s life. They had a funeral service for him in his beautiful garden on the lochside, and everyone turned out: we reckoned that when the first cars in the funeral procession were arriving here at the churchyard, the last ones were just leaving the farm. His widow has resisted the family's suggestions that she should move, still lives at the farm, doesn't drive, does bits and pieces about the place, and still talks of 'our' home.

I've often been struck by the element of romance surrounding A–'s death: died up on the hill, brought down by your son and your grandson, laid to rest by your wife, doctor makes tea for the family, funeral service in your garden surrounded by lifelong friends, everyone in the community pays their respects to you. I've talked a lot about the strength of the community here: there's no doubt in my mind that there's a spirit that binds all of us together and brings extra support to individuals and families (including ourselves) when times are hard. My patients, I think, see me as someone who'll attend to whatever needs to be done for them, whether it's complicated treatment or something much more mundane: terribly sort of Dr. Findlay's casebook – but it works!

12

Observations

There can be no doubt that the geographic, socio-economic and cultural profiles of communities are significant influences on the work of general practitioners, as are the personalities, professional interests and philosophies of health care of the GPs themselves. The consequence of this meshing of influences is that general practice, as seen in these examples from Scotland in the late 1990s, is a very diverse activity, with ill-defined boundaries. Diversity of activity and vagueness of boundaries are inevitable consequences of the definition of the GP as a medical generalist committed to the care of the whole person; such a commitment, however, is also responsible for the common ground, in terms of professional and personal pre-occupations and issues to be addressed, that can be identified among GPs working in very different settings.

The commitment to the whole person makes the work of general practice inherently problematic; because of it, GPs cannot necessarily identify or establish strict boundaries to intervention and responsibility. Nor can they be entirely objective or distance themselves completely from their patients' lives. Particularly in impoverished communities, caring for health involves dealing with a great deal of minor self-limiting illness compounded with the destructive effects on the individual of poverty and deprivation, of lack of hope and any sense of a better future. Nowhere, perhaps, are the influences of non-medical problems on personal notions of health and illness so clearly seen – and it is precisely here, despite the strong presence of other caring professionals offering support, that the doctor is the one, above all others, to whom people turn; the doctor is readily available, highly trusted, and will not turn you away.

While this is a very attractive arrangement for the patient, it can be a source of ethical dilemma for the GP; as has been recounted here, the non-medical problems which patients present can range from domestic violence to having a partner in police custody and wishing to have him released on medical grounds. In the former case, prescribing tranquillisers to women enduring violent relationships may at first seem like an unethical solution to the problem; the question arises, however, what else, in these situations, is the compassionate GP to do? Ideally, the 'treatment' would be to remove the cause of suffering, but clearly this is often not possible, which leaves the GP with a dilemma. As regards a patient asking a GP to use another patient's medical condition manipulatively, while this may seem reasonable to the patient, it is unlikely to be ethically defensible to the GP.

Health promotion programmes can also pose problems. That the level of prosperity of any community clearly has such a profound effect on health and illness would in itself suggest that monolithic 'health for all' campaigns and targets have little chance of universal success. As one GP working in a deprived area commented, many health promotion targets simply 'refer to a different population'. Here again doctors may be placed in a difficult and frustrating position through being asked to combine their realistic view of the possibility of change in a patient's unhealthy lifestyle with support for health targets (regarding, for example, smoking, alcohol consumption or healthy eating) which they know to be unattainable. The evidence would seem to suggest that a more subtle, personally relevant approach is needed; if general practice is intended to be patient centred then it must follow from that that agendas for health promotion should be tailored to fit individual communities.

It is clear that the wide variety of ways in which people turn to their GP extends the role well beyond actual medical knowledge, skills and interventions to embrace the concept of someone capable of just 'being there' in a time of crisis. A potent example of this is the involvement of GPs in terminal care and bereavement where medical expertise is willingly combined with simply being around to provide psychological and social support for patient and carers alike. That so many GPs identify terminal care as one of the most satisfying areas of general practice is indicative of widespread regard for this aspect of the work.

While the medical model at the heart of our current healthcare system is based on a mechanical view of human beings as bodies which can be broken up into component systems, one of the distinctive features of clinical care in general practice is the recognition of the close interplay of physical, psychological and social factors. The GP's generalist skills are not simply an amalgam of bits of other specialities such as surgery, medicine, paediatrics and gynaecology; they also include, along with knowledge of the latest drug treatments and investigations, the skill of integrating information derived from the patient's background and an appreciation of the patient's own perspective.

Given the wide demands made on GPs, how can they best be prepared for the job that lies ahead? It is probably the case that no one can be made completely aware, in advance, of what working as a GP will be like; nevertheless, in contrast to earlier situations where new GPs could be left feeling completely at sea, the recent development of structured post-graduate training has undoubtedly provided valuable learning opportunities. GP training schemes, however, are still largely about providing knowledge and skills in terms of traditional diagnostic approaches to patients' complaints; it may only be when the GP registrar has gained confidence in this decision-making, and in working knowledgeably with the vast array of drugs now available, that she or he can begin to think about the other knowledge and skills required. GPs undoubtedly also need to acquire a range of coping strategies which will allow them to survive the impact of around 6,000 unpredictable consultations a year; it is particularly in these areas of personal development that the role of trainers and other mentors in extending problem-solving skills, providing sounding boards and giving feedback, is invaluable.

Preparing for general practice has also to include knowledge and understanding of business management as development planning is, increasingly, a part of life for GPs. While some GPs feel that there's an over emphasis on the business side, it remains true that GPs are independent contractors organising health care running into millions of pounds; it would therefore be unwise to dismiss the importance of developing sound financial management skills. While fund-holding had a mixed press, there can be little doubt that it was a useful stimulus to many practices which were able, thereby, to define objectives, purchase care for groups of patients, and strengthen their practice teams.

The extent to which there have been winners and losers as regards fund-holding is difficult to assess as all views on the issue are to some extent subjective and dependent on differing philosophies of care. Achieving efficiency in future will, however, certainly mean the coming together of larger groups to share management costs and support staff. While the loss of smaller practices of two or three partners does seem inevitable, it is still regrettable as larger, more complex teams of providers may well deliver a less personal service to the patient.

Working in larger teams may, however, actually benefit doctors, both practically and educationally. Since doctors learn best from each other, the way in which groups of GPs working in the same practice can now identify and plan for their own training needs should be seen as a positive development. Information technology also has a part to play here, with e-mail and the internet providing enormous opportunities for home-based education. Doctors will however still need to meet together; it is unlikely, for example, that a computer will ever replace face to face discussion as the means of unravelling the feelings which inevitably arise from the very personal involvement with patients' difficulties which GPs experience.

How general practice should be structured has been continually debated throughout the 1990s. The organisation of medicine into bureaucratic systems with an inherent interest in efficiency does not necessarily appeal to doctors who cherish their clinical independence; some feel that conglomerates, consortia and health maintenance organisations may, in the end, deliver a service which is consistent but unimaginative. The fear in some quarters is that such organisations will result in assembly-line medicine where patient-centredness becomes subordinate to computer-based disease-centred approaches. Such a system might work efficiently enough for a limited number of problems, and even seem better (for those situations) than the sometimes apparently inefficient, personalised care currently offered; despite the current pre-occupation with molecular biology as the centre point of advances in medical care, however, illness itself continues to be unorganised. The challenge for the future is how we cope with this.

GPs do think of themselves as caring people and as both doctors and citizens generally feel a commitment to handling the huge variety of complex problems with which they are presented. There is a growing realisation, however, that while the breadth of general practice is a core strength it may also be a weakness. In an open-access service which is demand led, there are many different issues at the forefront of care: birth control, genetic manipulation, euthanasia, physical disease, poverty, nourishment, psychological problems, narcotics and accidents are just a few of these. With so vast a list of competing issues already before them, many doctors are now urging resistance to efforts to push the boundaries of general practice even further. Their argument is that it is inappropriate for them to embrace ever-increasing social problems, or identify deprived children and unsatisfactory parents, or badger housing departments, or monitor truancy – all on the pretext of caring for the whole person. Perhaps, in order to survive, GPs will, in future, have to disavow responsibility for some kinds of problems.

So what is the solution to the problems of roles and pressure and boundaries which general practitioners now face? In the accounts of general practice given here, the growing importance of teamwork is constantly emphasised; even now, nurses, health visitors, community psychiatric nurses and a whole range of other health care professionals – including social workers and counsellors – all play a significant and increasing part in primary care. Rightly so, some might say, because for some aspects of general practice – dealing, for example, with the large volume of self-limiting minor illness or stress or essentially practical problems that patients present – it has to be asked whether, in terms of cost-benefit and the judicious spending of public money, an expensively-trained GP is always the right person to be doing the problem-solving. For any team to work effectively however, roles, responsibilities and status must be made clear and the needs of individuals and sub-groups identified. One difficulty currently facing general practice is that while it is acknowledged that many of the tasks traditionally undertaken by doctors can be successfully delegated to other team members, the status of doctors in any team remains significantly higher than that of others. Questions of which professionals might, in future, lead multi-disciplinary primary care teams, likewise remain unresolved.

The work of general practice is undoubtedly stressful; interrupted sleep, lack of regular working hours and the fatiguing effect of an unending stream of patients' 'stories' all drain time and energy. The medical profession has a tendency to expect its practitioners to be superhuman; with the stresses of life as a GP now being more openly discussed, however, many younger doctors are less willing to sign up for traditional partnership arrangements which they know will involve significant personal sacrifice in the interests of patient care. Traditionalists see this as a lack of commitment, but it has to be recognised that, even with the advent of GP deputising services (which generally work well) life as a GP is hugely demanding in terms of hours and responsibilities. The relentless drain on time inherent in full-time GP work also raises important questions regarding equal opportunity; women now constitute 50% of medical graduates, and for those who wish to combine career and family it can be, at present, very difficult to find satisfying work. How, in future, we optimise the contribution of women is a challenge to the profession.

The foregoing accounts of general practice speak for themselves. The work of general practitioners is not just one other branch of professional life; it also provides, in the nature of the interactions with individual, family and community, one of the most powerful immediate reflections of the state of society available to us. It is significant that some of the GPs interviewed for this book identify the best means of improving the health of the nation not as pouring ever-increasing sums of money into the NHS itself, but rather as providing significantly increased investment in housing, employment, education and training. Such an identification of significant environmental influences on health, made by GPs themselves, merits a response; it derives, after all, from first-hand knowledge of people's lives. Until the health issues linked to deprivation are addressed, at least some of the vast sums of money sucked into health provision will have been spent in vain, because the difficulties of living in deprived communities not only increase ill-health through poor diet and low self-esteem, but all stress is magnified, resulting in many people enduring life-situations or acting in ways which are, in health terms, counter-productive.

Other significant influences on health and on the work of GPs are also touched on in the foregoing chapters – the effects of media coverage of medical issues; the demise of the extended family; the isolation of single parents, immigrant women and elderly people; the increasing pressure on the parents of very young children to go out to work; the spread of alcoholism and other drug addiction; the reluctance to take advantage of health screening and health services for adults and children, are just some of these. There are, in addition, glimpses of less widely known stresses which people endure, most hauntingly perhaps the stress of bereaved families who cannot easily grieve publicly because of the perceived shamefulness of a young person's death.

While there are many problems discussed in these pages, it would be wrong to allow them to completely overshadow the very positive and rewarding experiences which are also recorded. These can perhaps best be summed up as a deep feeling of satisfaction and purpose in the work, combined with the sense of pleasure and privilege in usefully belonging to a community where patients and doctor have a strong sense of mutual respect, and can even, at times, offer mutual support. The commitment of the GPs interviewed here is reassuringly strong and the frank accounts of personal journeys in medicine both illuminating and moving. The next fifty years will be an interesting time for our health service; in the view of many, it will either fragment into rationalised, competent, managed care systems where doctors clock on and off, or something quite different, which continues to acknowledge the value of all three 'C's – compassion and continuity of care as well as competence – will emerge. If the latter does happen the role of the practitioner who, as here, virtuously combines scientific knowledge with 'healing' arts, may still be secure.